STRETCH

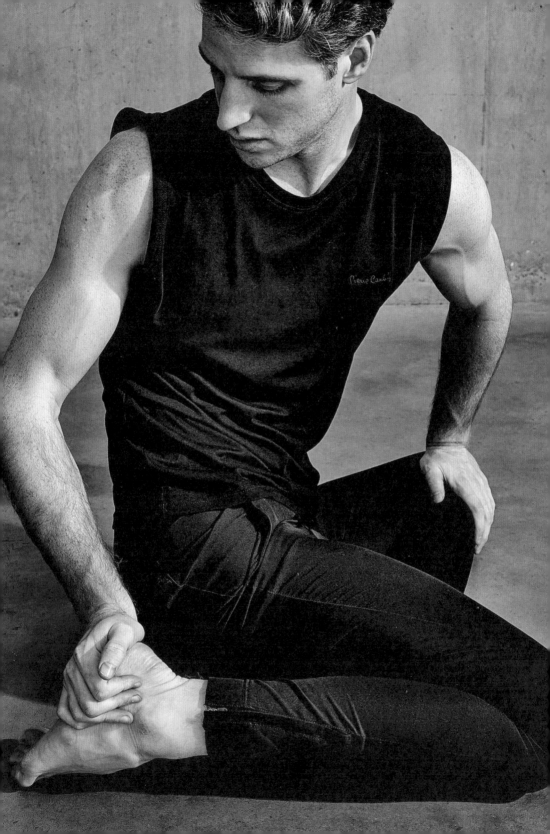

ROGER FRAMPTON

STRETCH

SEVEN DAILY MOVEMENTS TO SET YOUR BODY FREE

PAVILION

CONTENTS

INTRODUCTION

As adults we are often in awe of babies and young children who bend, squat and roll around with ease. These effortless movements go way beyond the fact that babies are born with more bones and soft cartilage than adults. If that were true, flexibility and mobility would be impossible for adults. Similarly, if you travel from the West to other parts of the world, particularly Africa and Asia, you'll notice not just children but adults, often even the elderly, sitting in a squat position with comfort and ease. These simple movements performed on a daily basis help to keep people mobile and flexible into old age. In contrast, our mostly sedentary Western culture, where we often move from sitting in an office chair all day to the sofa in front of the TV in the evening, has resulted in us losing our flexibility – a choice for which we're paying an expensive and painful price.

Since becoming a qualified coach in 2011, I have focused on how to improve natural movement, targeting the root of the problem to give your body long-lasting mobility. The Frampton Method uses conscious movement, combining bodyweight exercises with aspects of gymnastics and yoga to better help us understand the natural functionality of the body. When that happens, you decrease the likelihood of injuries, chronic pain and other spine-associated issues that hinder health by learning how to move instead of obsessing over how much you move. The Frampton Method ensures that you move with purpose and precision, increasing the chance of recovery and prevention of injury as well as common aches and pains.

Natural movement, with a series of stretches, has been proven to benefit your overall long-term health, from increasing blood flow to joints and muscles to improving balance and breathing. Furthermore, the best part is that it doesn't even require a gym membership. *Stretch* takes you back to the basics, guiding you through a daily routine to regain essential lost movements. It includes seven principle stretches (with variations on each stretch) designed to improve everyday movement. Each exercise takes a minute to perform and can be practised at any time, in any place. These movements focus on the critical areas of the body, namely: the **spine**, **hips** and **shoulders**, as well as **balance**, which is essential to your overall and long-term mobility.

THE SEVEN ESSENTIAL MOVEMENTS ARE:

1. **SPINE ROTATION**

2. **SPINE EXTENSION**

3. **SPINE FLEXION**

4. **LATERAL FLEXION**

5. **HIP MOBILITY**

6. **SHOULDER ROTATION**

7. **BALANCE**

So that is:

**4 x spine, 1 x hips, 1 x shoulders and 1 x balance
= 7 essential stretches.**

Try to remember this phrase. You'll be using this every day to form the habits that will take care of your long-term mobility.

I look at agility and mobility as akin to brushing your teeth twice a day. With this daily programme of seven simple movements, your muscles will start relaxing and your posture will become less rigid – it has never been easier to combat the common aches and pains acquired through too much sitting. The trick is to stay consistent and committed to the seven movements and remember that these routines are not a quick fix that will transform your body overnight. These are habits you are forming for life!

IT'S TIME TO STRETCH!

HOW

WE MOVE

HOW MUCH WE MOVE VS HOW WE MOVE

Whether you have done your steps today or not we've all heard the question, 'Have you done your steps today?' and there are several reasons why. While recent research has traced the origin of the '10,000 steps per day' goal to a Japanese marketing slogan for a step counter, the catchy marketing gimmick subsequently morphed into a fitness mantra which helped kick-start the 'move more' movement. Since then, scientific studies have supported the 'move more' theory, with some showing that participants managed to control their diabetes or cholesterol levels better when increasing their daily step count.

There are numerous health benefits to be gained by moving often throughout the day, including lowering your blood pressure, stabilizing your blood sugar and reducing your risk of a heart attack. So, we all know that we are supposed to move more and many of us even possess some sort of wearable tech to track the distance we cover. However, it seems that while we can agree that how *much* we move is important, *how* we actually move is still somewhat ignored.

We blindly set ourselves on the wrong course of action when we focus *just* on movement instead of *natural* movement. With the right techniques and returning to our natural movement, we can not only lead healthier and more active lives, but we can perhaps also avoid spending our later years in excruciating pain or dependency due to immobility.

The next step to a long-term mobile body is to start to move it as it evolved to move or, for want of a better phrase, as it 'should'. I say 'should' because the body can move in a multitude of different ways. In this book, I want to take you on a journey back in time via the evolution of mankind to the seven movements that make up the essence of human movement. On the road to getting your natural movement back, it is essential that you spend some time undoing the tightness that previous inactivity has caused and start moving again at your full range of capacity.

Many of us are stuck in a cycle of pain – tight shoulders, bad backs, stiff necks – simply because we're not moving as we should be. Due to the sedentary nature of modern life, the unfortunate destiny for the majority of people is muscles and joints that slowly tighten over the years as we endlessly sit down in chairs. If we don't use the full capacity of our bodies, we start to lose it, and then one day we realize that we can't do the natural movements we could easily perform as children – like sitting comfortably in a squat position, touching our toes or sitting upright on the floor. Our bodies have lost their basic primal movements.

INSTINCTIVE MOVEMENT

All animals, humans included, teach themselves how to move. I think there is a common misconception that our parents teach us how to walk, perhaps because they stand next to us ready to catch us when we fall, trying to minimize how much we hurt ourselves. But if you really think about it logically, children learning to move aren't actually copying their parents. Children sit bolt upright on the floor, put their toes in their mouths and palms on the ground. I think we can agree that an extremely large percentage of parents would fail to copy one, if any, of those movements.

Natural movement is not a learned behaviour but rather intuitive, genetic and part of our human code. The reason I really need you to know this is so you realize that you are not genetically inflexible. Of course, some people are more inherently flexible than others, but we all start out with the same bendy bodies. Perhaps you're strong and fit now or perhaps you've been doing a specific sport or spent a lot of time static, sitting in school chairs and at work desks and you've lost some of that flexibility, but it's important to know that we all started out the same – with free-moving bodies.

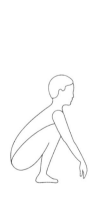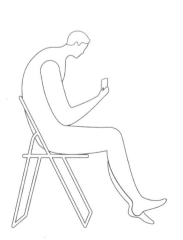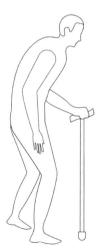

WHERE DOES IT ALL GO WRONG?

The illustration opposite represents the human cycle of movement from childhood through to old age. Part 2 of the cycle is where we start to lose our innate flexibility and a whole host of things begin to go against us, including the biggest killer of instinctive movement: society.

Why would a child who is squatting naturally to pick things up from the floor suddenly stop? Why would a child who is moving through numerous bodily positions start to lose the natural movement they begin life with? I'm going to break down what I believe to be are two of the biggest causes:

1 The first cause that we cannot ignore is our education system. In the UK, especially, we have a school system which includes A LOT of repetitive sitting down. I'm not taking anything away from how important and fundamental our education system is, but we can't turn a blind eye to the fact that kids are taught to sit on a chair for five hours a day. An Australian study tested kids' behaviour when given the option of using a sit-to-stand desk. The good news is that when given the option of these different desks, kids use them. A step in the right direction.

2 The second biggest cause is mimicking. Children navigate the world by mimicking the adults around them. It's not only language they learn from their parents, but those hours spent sitting on a sofa watching TV or working at a desk are also being mimicked daily. We are the example they are learning from, whether we are doing something that we want them to copy or not.

If children don't see adults doing any form of movement practice, they see it as normal that they don't either, or that sport is just for kids. We can send them off to all the sports in the world, but if they watch us indulging in work, Netflix and sofa-slouching with no time dedicated to undoing some of the tightness caused by that, then that is the message that will stay with them. When they become an adult, that is the behaviour they will mimic. Kids copy what they see, rather than what we tell them to do. They are much more likely to move intuitively and respect their bodies' natural movement if they see the adults around them doing the same.

This is why, when parents come to me and ask: 'What can I do to make sure my kid moves the best?', I say, 'lead by example'. In fact, my TED talk ended with this statement: 'We should lead by example and move like them'. And where should we start with that? Right where we began. By integrating the essential stretches into our lives and regaining full access to our bodies.

MOVE IT
OR LOSE IT

Whatever we practise, we get better at. If we run all the time, we become better at running, if we swim or cycle consistently, our bodies adapt to help us become better at those activities. However, the problem with all this is that, if we only improve the skills that we practise, then the opposite also applies – the skills we don't practise, we lose. Our body is an energy-efficient machine that does not waste its capacity keeping hold of skills that we no longer require. Why should it? The body focuses its efforts on what is required or what is practised. So, you shouldn't be *that* surprised if you can't touch your toes.

While your body is busy learning new skills and postures, such as hunching over a phone or laptop, it's also busy forgetting the skills that it doesn't deem necessary, like squatting. It makes sense when we think about it in terms of evolution. When food and survival were top of the agenda, the last thing we wanted was for our body to use up all of its resources maintaining skills it doesn't use. Your brain doesn't have a long-term plan. It focuses on the present – mainly food and procreation – so it can't really be trusted to be in charge of your long-term health.

Modern medicine has done some amazing things for the human species. For example, we are living longer than ever before, which sounds great in theory. However, what's the point of living to a record age when you then spend many of those extra years frozen in an armchair, unable to take care of yourself, let alone anyone around you? Wouldn't it be wonderful if we could live to a ripe old age AND still be able to be an engaged part of the community, instead of relegated to an armchair? The good news is that it's never too late.

The common narrative is that, as we get older, we should 'slow down'. However, if you've read my first book, *The Flexible Body*, you'll know that I disagree. I'm a big believer in the 'move it or lose it' theory, which says that when we stop using a movement, we lose that movement.

FOR EXAMPLE:

+ Stop sitting in a squat = lose the ability to sit in a squat
+ Stop folding down to touch our toes = maintain the tightness of the legs and back of the body

Now, these examples may seem very simple but, when we take them further, the comparisons become a little more extreme:

+ Stop taking the stairs = lose the ability to walk up a flight of stairs
+ Stop walking regularly = lose the ability to walk
+ Rely on our arms to get out of the armchair = lose the ability to use our hips to stand up

The above statements may seem a little dramatic but for a large number of elderly people, this is a living reality. It's essential that we constantly come up with ways that keep us moving. Walking is a good start, but we also need activities to get our bodies moving in ALL directions, which is why I recommend living in a house with stairs whenever possible. You never want to limit your options for movement but instead look for ways in which you can make good movement part of your daily habits. The short-term brain wants to make life convenient, the long-term moving body needs us to challenge our movement on a daily basis.

GETTING OUR FLEXIBILITY BACK

Several years ago, I was sitting in a gymnastics class, scratching my head thinking – how did I become so inflexible? The coach, Alex, was showing a group of us how to do a bridge. He wasn't demonstrating himself however, his little six-year-old assistant was doing it for him, effortlessly and happily. We all looked at each other and smiled as if to say, 'OK, just like that then?'.

After the class, I spoke to Alex and asked, 'What should I be working on if I want to be able to do the exercises more easily?'. His reply was pretty direct: 'You're just tight mate, you need to get some of that flexibility back'. 'Back?!' As far as I was concerned, or could remember, I'd never been able to touch my toes, sit in a squat or even to sit comfortably on the floor without my knees hurting, or my back rounding.

I didn't know it at the time, but I'd just had a pivotal conversation. It marked the beginning of something not only special and life-changing for me personally, but that literally millions of people around the world would eventually hear me speak about in my TED talk.

I was a fit but very stiff guy (who aspired to be like Arnold Schwarzenegger) who realized in a gym class that he'd unwittingly sacrificed the primal movements he had started life with. From that day on my life changed. I started to understand what Alex meant by getting it 'back'. I suddenly began to notice little kids in the park, on the street and in cafés, sitting and playing happily in a squat position. Completely perfect squats with their feet straight and their backs like iron rods. He was right, we all start out flexible! These little humans were geniuses at movement.

Nearly all of us have gone through this same journey towards inflexibility – which I call the movement cycle (explained on pages 13) – but the good news is it can be easily reversed.

STRETCHING? BUT THAT'S JUST WARM-UP EXERCISES, RIGHT?

When I explain my coaching methods, it always pains me to hear this common misconception. Stretching has for too long been thought of as something that happens for 30 seconds before or after a workout.

I want to shine some light on stretching from a different perspective. In my view, stretching my body IS my workout. I'm not talking here about a relaxed 30 seconds, but a focused practice based on regaining my natural movement. Not only is it a workout but it's my most essential workout because, if my body is tight, I'm not using it to its full capacity.

Tightness in the body forces you to move in ways you are not supposed to. It puts unnecessary pressure on your spine, wrecks your hips and shoulders and prevents you from doing basic tasks without the onset of pain.

Many of us have lost access to the majority of our body and are suffering the everyday consequences in the form of back pain, neck ache and postural issues, simply because we've become too tight. That's right, you're in a body right this very second that you don't have full access to. Imagine what could be possible when you gain more access to it.

Let's look at a hypothetical sliding scale of how our range of movement can decline with age. This is a very loose average – in the UK, for example, there would be a much steeper decline than in countries where it's socially acceptable for groups of elderly people to dance in the parks.

I want you to take a moment and consider what range of movement you have access to? Be real with yourself and have an honest conversation. Are you moving well for your age or could you be doing more? Where is it that you want to end up? Do you want to work with me, starting from today, to take those essential steps to get your natural movement back?

The aim of this exercise is not to scare you but to be realistic about how life is for a large number of people. However, you should know that there are many examples of 90-year-olds having better access to their bodies than ten-year-olds. There's nothing to say you can't be one of them!

'But isn't it natural for our bodies to decline as we age?' This is the classic question I get as soon as I discuss gaining better range of movement as we age. Of course, as we get older we do slow down. However, I am saying that it is possible to reverse this chart, it's just that most people aren't prepared to put in small efforts every day for the later reward. It takes discipline to be able to do that and, if you speak to any elderly person who is disciplined enough to do what it takes, I bet my bottom dollar they will all give you a similar answer as to how they do it – you just get on with it. No matter if you're having a bad day, no matter if you're tired or busy. It's 1 per cent of your day and you have to take responsibility and get this done for the sake of your future self.

1-YEAR-OLD – 100 PER CENT ACCESS
(MOVING IN A HUGE VARIETY OF SHAPES ALL DAY LONG)

10-YEAR-OLD – 95 PER CENT ACCESS

20-YEAR-OLD – 90 PER CENT ACCESS

30-YEAR-OLD – 85 PER CENT ACCESS

40-YEAR-OLD – 80 PER CENT ACCESS

50-YEAR-OLD – 75 PER CENT ACCESS

60-YEAR-OLD – 70 PER CENT ACCESS

70-YEAR-OLD – 65 PER CENT ACCESS

80-YEAR-OLD – 60 PER CENT ACCESS

90-YEAR-OLD – 50 PER CENT ACCESS
(VERY LIMITED MOVEMENT)

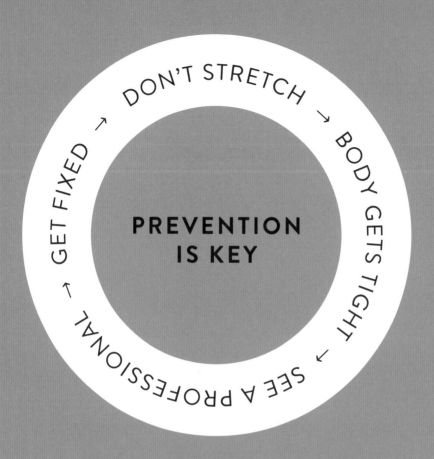

DON'T STRETCH → BODY GETS TIGHT → SEE A PROFESSIONAL → GET FIXED →

PREVENTION IS KEY

The biggie right here is the 'don't stretch' part. We could also say it's the 'don't take responsibility' part. Unlike other things in life, movement isn't something somebody else can do for you. You can get the best coaches, apps and programmes in the world but it's you who has to do the work. There isn't any way around this and the buck stops with you.

But people do believe they can somehow get around this. It's like saying, 'I'm not going to brush my teeth but I'm going to see the hygienist twice a year'. It doesn't work – and the biggest reason I know it doesn't work? Because I see the same messages from people no matter the professional they see: 'I went to the chiropractor and they told me this.' 'I went to the physio and he told me this'. Now, I'm not saying what they've told you isn't true, but I am saying that you can't sit in a chair for nine hours a day, not do any preventative work and complain to a physio when you feel pain. We often wait for a problem to pop up and then see a professional, as opposed to avoiding the cause by having a regular movement practice that takes care of the body's needs.

I could liken this to not servicing your car and waiting until you break down. Brush your teeth twice a day and your teeth won't rot – stretching your body daily is nothing more than necessary physical hygiene.

Just because it's the social norm *not* to stretch daily and then complain to a professional when your body has taken enough of your crap, why accept it just because everyone else is doing it? Why not be inspired by the few – people in their sixties, seventies, eighties and even nineties – doing what it takes to prove to the younger ones, that it's possible and requires nothing more than a little bit of daily discipline – just 1 per cent of your waking day. We've got to stop looking outside of ourselves for the fix.

> We taught ourselves how to move, we've incurred the damage and we must take responsibility and undo it, ourselves.

I was tighter at 22 than I am now at the time of writing this, which is 36. In 14 years, I've flipped the chart on its head. I am certainly not somebody you would say is 'naturally flexible'. I was told by a chiropractor that my spine was 'twisted' and by a physio that I had 'short hamstrings'. Luckily, I learned at a young age not to pay too much attention to what appear to be shortcomings and focused my mind on what I wanted.

It can be extremely easy to find something 'wrong' with you, but the truth is, it's not very helpful and, no matter which professional you see, you'll probably get a different story. The point is to focus your attention on what it is you want to achieve. If you like, you can copy my belief that I can achieve anything I want in my life and with my body. This works for me and I find anyone who says any different to be quite strange and odd; 'I'm sorry, my friend, you must be confused. My body is a phenomenal machine that can achieve feats that haven't even been discovered yet.' I focus my attention on the people who are leading the way and strongly suggest you do the same. You will find that these are the people who have worked hard to get their bodies to the place they want them to be. When you start, all you need is that tiny bit of evidence that you can regain some of your natural movement and suddenly you see how practice works and how your consistency adds up, just as with any skill. Like learning a new language, it seems a daunting task from the outset but, as soon as you get into that flow, it will become a habit.

IS SITTING DOWN DESTROYING ME?

Guilty! I did name my TED talk 'Why sitting down destroys you', but I have a very valid point. The idea that repetitive sitting is severely damaging to our long-term health became popular when health practitioners and fitness experts started to look at the disadvantages of long hours of sitting down. Dr James A. Levine proclaiming 'sitting is the new smoking' was a stroke of genius. It indicated that we were once again subjecting ourselves to poor health through a preventable cause; in this case sitting.

However, the idea of leaving behind our chair-centric lifestyle is more challenging than quitting smoking. Not only are architects inclined to create space for sitting arrangements in any building they design, but most jobs require us to spend a substantial amount of time sitting at a desk.

In England alone, an average employee spends approximately 9.5 hours per day sedentary. This only increases as we age. Seniors aged 65–74 spend more than 10 hours per day sitting. That means 75 per cent of our waking hours are spent either in a chair or some other passive mode (slouching on a sofa, for example).

Countless research has proved the harmful effects of sitting and these studies aren't just restricted to corporate workers. The NHS discovered a 'link between illness and sitting' dating back to the 1950s. A comparative analysis of bus drivers and conductors concluded that the drivers had a higher chance of developing heart problems than their colleagues. Results indicated that excessive sitting might cause 'weaker muscles and bones'. [1] The British Heart Foundation states that: 'Compared to people who sit the least, people who sit for prolonged hours have a higher risk of contracting fatal and chronic diseases.'

Further research reveals that too much sitting can lead to:

- 112 per cent increased risk of diabetes

- 147 per cent increased risk of cardiovascular events, like heart attack and stroke

- 90 per cent increased risk of death from cardiovascular events

This is just the tip of the iceberg as the other parts of the body are also affected by our chair-loving habits. Our posture, for instance, is being distorted due to corporate hours designated to the desk. Back in 2016, the British Chiropractic Association (BCA) discovered that more than 41 per cent of workers suffer from back and neck pain, predominantly caused by sitting in one place for extended periods. [2] These numbers have increased drastically due to the 2020 pandemic, with a huge number of people having to work from home, confined to their houses without access to gyms or other means of exercise (see pages 24–26 for more on what you can do combat the effects of home working).

[1] https://www.nhs.uk/live-well/exercise/why-sitting-too-much-is-bad-for-us/
[2] https://chiropractic-uk.co.uk/uk-risk-back-health-when-working-from-home/

SITTING IS THE NEW SMOKING

WORKING FROM HOME

As we move deeper into the digital age, where more of us are working from home, it's now more essential than ever that we give our bodies the movement that they deserve. 2020 will be the year none of us will ever forget. For many, it meant a huge transition to working from home; but how has this affected our movement? Interestingly, when we were told we could only leave the house for an hour a day, it made some people exercise who, in normal circumstances, would not. Suddenly, walking became the most important thing and proved our essential need to move our bodies on a daily basis.

Pandemic aside, working from home is becoming the norm for many of us and this presents a whole new array of bonuses for incorporating better movement into our lives. I want you to embrace it and all the free-moving benefits it can offer. Below are some of my suggestions for best work-from-home practice from movement to taking time out.

ARE YOU SITTING COMFORTABLY?

One of the ways we can stop postural issues which inevitably lead to pain points is to be aware of our bodies when we are sitting or standing. When you're working from home, you can work standing, sitting on the floor, even lying on your front on the floor. No-one is around so you don't have to feel like the odd one out. You can give your body a whole new range of positions as opposed to one static one in a chair. Variety really is the key.

The illustrations opposite show you some sitting positions that I use on a daily basis and all you need is a short table, such as a coffee table. Sitting upright against a wall really helps to keep the back straighter. Using blocks and books to sit on is also an option. I advise positioning yourself so that your eye line is level with the top of the laptop screen.

If floor-based working isn't a realistic option for you here are my two biggest tips for working at a desk which will make a significant impact on your life and also triple your progress when it comes to stretching the body. Because, why do all the good work undoing our bodies from tightness only to continue with our postural habits and retighten the body up again.

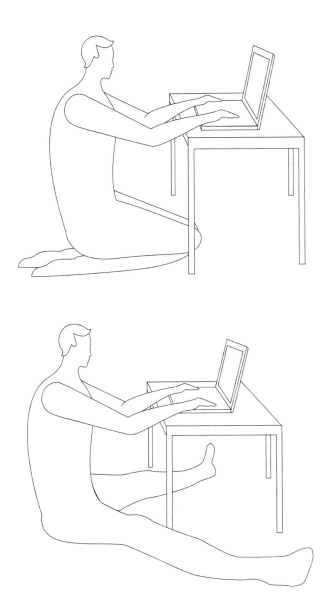

1 **Uncross everything** – those feet, those arms, those legs. Constant crossing (because it's always on the same side), will literally twist your body into pain points. Look, I know it's comfortable, but it's a habit, a habit that by breaking will eliminate that tight side, and the other areas it's affecting for good.

2 **The Goldilocks moment** – not too tense, not too relaxed but something in the middle. In order to combat slouching we are lead to believe we must sit bolt upright all day long. Not only is this exhausting, it's unrealistic. The opposite is also true, slouching will lead to rounded spines and a forward head posture. Think about Goldilocks – not too tense, equally not too relaxed, but holding yourself with a constant awareness of the position of your body.

TAKE A BREAK

Have you ever spent the morning so engrossed in e-mails or phone calls that, when you look up, you realize 3 hours have passed? It is all too easy to lose track of time when working from home. This is where the seven daily movements come in. I encourage you to build in a movement schedule that works for you and fit it around your working day.

Try a simple stretch, such as the Sofa Extension (page 68), as soon as you wake up, practise the Door Frame Stretch (page 92) whilst you wait for the kettle to boil, and why not spend the afternoon working in one of the positions illustrated on the previous page? If you're not spending as much time commuting to and from work, you can use that time for other activities that are essential to your long-term health. Make sure you are not just filling that gap with more screen time and entertainment but instead focusing on something which will provide long-term satisfaction and rewards. Sitting on a comfy couch is just as detrimental as those office chairs, but by dedicating some time each day to stretch you will begin to form a good habit. This in turn will make it easier to remain consistent as it becomes second nature.

PRIORITIZING CONSCIOUS MOVEMENT

The human brain is wired for instant gratification. Our brains prioritize the thing that offers the most instantaneous reward, which is why scrolling on social media seems a more attractive proposition than replying to all of those emails. We know stretching is good for us, but if we don't actually enjoy it, it's extremely challenging to get ourselves to actually do it.

Why is it that, no matter how much we want to, we find it so hard to prioritize the very things that are good for our long-term health? Like stretching. We know we should stretch, we know how to stretch, we know we don't need any equipment and we know that we are capable of doing it on our own. So, now we've ticked off the most common excuses for not doing it: what is the psychology behind it?

The sole reason that I have made progress with my flexibility (and I still have a way to go) is because I prioritize it. I schedule it like any other meeting. If I have a busy day, I will purposely write it in my diary to make sure that I tick it off for the day (see page 51 for our sample timetable). If I don't, it will just get lost or become the thing that there wasn't time for. It really doesn't matter when you do it. But it does matter that you do it.

For me, training is my reward and I try to look forward to it – I know that when I stretch it not only makes my body feel free but it has a direct impact on all other aspects of my life. I'm more focused at work, I sleep better, I make better decisions and I have more energy throughout the day.

I want you to feel the same way about it too and I want you to feel these benefits! The hardest part is starting – doing that first stretch – it may not be the most entertaining activity in the world but the more you do it, the more you'll see the benefits and the more you'll want to do it. Get it in your diary... today!

HOW TO

STRETCH

WHAT IS STRETCHING?

Before we get to the stretches, let's get back to basics and think about what you are really doing when you're stretching. When we stretch, we are lengthening or elongating.

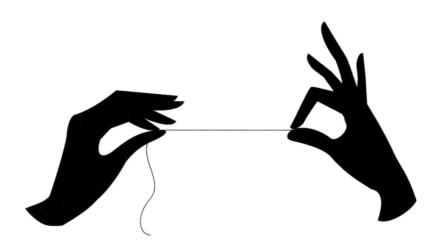

For this exercise, I want you to pick up the wire of your phone charger. (If you haven't already done so, then please unplug it!) Can you see how it's a bit 'slack'? Hold the wire with two fingers at one end and two fingers at the opposite end and very softly pull the wire taut. While looking at the wire, keep changing slowly between slack and taut. How many forces are making the wire straight?

The reason you're able to get the wire completely straight is that there are two forces pulling it in opposite directions. Now, pick up one end of the wire with one hand and lift it to the highest point you can while leaving the other end of the wire on the ground.

You can see you are stretching the wire but not quite to its full length. You would never be able to pull the wire to its full length with just one hand, unless the wire was heavier, and then you could use the force of gravity to lengthen it. To stretch the body fully, you need two forces pulling in opposite directions, just as with the wire you need two hands pulling at opposite ends to create maximum length.

From now on, think of your body as that wire – when you stretch it, you want to apply not one but two forces in opposite directions to get the most out of your stretches. Every single stretch in this book uses two forces. Keep asking in every stretch, 'what is the opposite force that I need to bring in here?' and always think about which area of the body you should be pushing and which part you should be pulling. When you get this right, you are stretching your body into its most lengthened state.

PLAY WITH YOUR EXERCISES

What are exercises? An exercise is either a position or a shape of the body, or a movement between a number of positions. There are millions of different exercises, plus all the variations with weights, sticks, blocks, on walls, on floors, standing, sitting, lying down, using furniture, on bars, on poles, in straps ... the list goes on! The exercise is merely a shape or a position. What you feel in that position is what determines whether you feel the exercise is 'the best thing since sliced bread' or 'this exercise doesn't work / is bad for me'.

Truth be told, neither is true. Exercises aren't 'amazing' and nor are they 'bad for you' – exercises should be played with. There are so many variants at play in an exercise that it's impossible to rule out the exercise before really breaking down every single moving part. If you get one part out of sync, or you lack a bit of tension in another, the exercise becomes a 'bad' exercise that doesn't work for you. However, if you adjust it slightly, that same exercise turns into a really strong stretch.

What we have to have in place is something called 'variants'. Exercises MUST be played with and explored. This is where you will get rewards.

Your mindset has an important role to play when doing the exercises. If you expect that the exercises in this book will be a 'perfect' fit for you and yet, as soon as you feel any discomfort, assume that it's a bad exercise, then you need to understand variants. You've got to be able to improvise, to listen to your body, to react to what comes up, to not throw your toys out of the pram and blame the exercise but instead ask yourself these questions:

'How can I make this exercise work for me?'

'Oh, I'm feeling discomfort when I do this; interesting, that's a message from my body. Let's play with some variants.'

'I don't feel anything here. What can I do to create more stretch?'

Your body is unique, made up of your daily postural habits, the positions you hold yourself in, the sports you've done, the chairs that you sit on, the way that you walk. These will all play a huge role in how the stretches in this book work for you.

WHAT ARE VARIANTS?

A variant is a minuscule change in angle within an exercise. To explain, let's take a look at a specific exercise in this book.

I'm performing 'Sitting Side Stretch' and I just can't feel a stretch. Instead of saying, 'This exercise isn't right for me', we need to try variants. We're not 'changing' the exercise but rather looking for ways to make the exercise work for you.

Push through the shoulder / relax the shoulder
Drop the front knee forwards / open the front knee wide
Try hip on the floor / off the floor
Bring the hand closer to me / further from me
Pull the ribs in / push the ribs open

And just like that, we have 10 new ways to make the exercise work for us. Can you see how, in each movement option, there was also an opposite? Exploring each of the stretches is going to be key to your progress.

STRETCHING TECHNIQUES

'Should I stay still or move within the stretch?' is a very common and important question, so let's go a bit deeper into why I use static or slow movement in my exercises.

When I first began my career as a movement coach, I actually started off teaching faster movements, such as the everyday exercises you come across in the fitness industry – lunges, squats, push-ups etc. But then I noticed how, when different people were doing the same exercise, they didn't look the same. When I looked more closely at how people were performing their exercises, I started to notice huge flaws. It wasn't that they were 'doing it wrong', but they were moving so fast that it just wasn't possible to pay full attention to the details of the exercise.

For example, if you're learning to run, you don't just run as fast as you can over and over again and expect to be a great runner. You have to break down the details – the foot position, the stride length, the body position, what the hands are doing, how high the knees come up. These are all crucial and, if you don't get these aspects right, you're not going to be able to run as efficiently as somebody who takes the time to learn the details. This takes dedication, practice and repetition.

But, for some reason, the fitness industry is different. It's a big free-for-all where everyone is trying to mimic professional athletes with no regard for the detail and technique involved. They just jump on a treadmill and wonder why, a few months later, their knee is in agony. This is a recipe for injuries and trips to the physio. It's like giving a toddler an exam paper – the paper will get some pen on it, but it will be a big mess.

Once I started to see this, I began to slow everything down. Not only with the people I was teaching but also in my own training. When you start to see the world in slow motion, you begin to see things that you never noticed before. Moving at a faster pace has benefits for cardiovascular fitness but, in terms of improving mobility and flexibility, it doesn't work. These exercises need to be performed at a pace that allows you to pay full attention to your whole body. The speed will come later, but only as you improve on the technique.

In all the stretches I am either still or moving slowly because I believe that, when we're training, we should give our bodies the full attention that they deserve. I only teach and perform slow movement so that I can be truly aware of all the parts of our body. The best way to see the detail in exercises and to be sure you're doing them correctly is to be still. When you freeze the frame you can't go wrong; you can pay attention to the position of your feet, your toes and your joints and then you'll realize that all of these moving parts have an effect. If you get the foot position wrong, then that will have a detrimental effect on the hips and vice versa. It's only through being still that you can truly see how that position feels for you.

So, is this static stretching? Well, the position at the beginning of the stretch should be different to the position at the end, so if you're further into the stretch by the end, it definitely isn't static. Let's look at an example:

Stand up wherever you are and relax down to touch your toes, keeping your legs straight and feet hip-width apart. Be aware of exactly how far you are into the stretch at the beginning. Then put a timer on your phone and see where you are after 30 seconds. Are you further? Maybe, maybe not. Try it for 1 minute, then 2 minutes, 3 minutes and 5 minutes. All I want you to do is to notice if there is a change. Really try to relax your torso when you do this.

You will see some kind of difference throughout the time and that difference will increase the more you perform the stretch. Soon, the position you achieved by the 3-minute mark will be your starting position. Now, before you say that's a long time to stay in a stretch, you can probably guess my answer. We can't complain about being in a stretch for 5 minutes when we happily sit in the same position at a desk for several hours!

But that does raise the question – how long should I stay in the stretches in this book? I suggest starting off with 1 minute, using either slow movement within the stretch or staying still. However, try not to have this time stuck in your head or obsess over it. If all you're thinking about is the time, then you've missed the point of stretching. It's about listening to your body, acknowledging how it feels and reacting accordingly. The length of the stretch is not what makes you progress; it's doing it repeatedly.

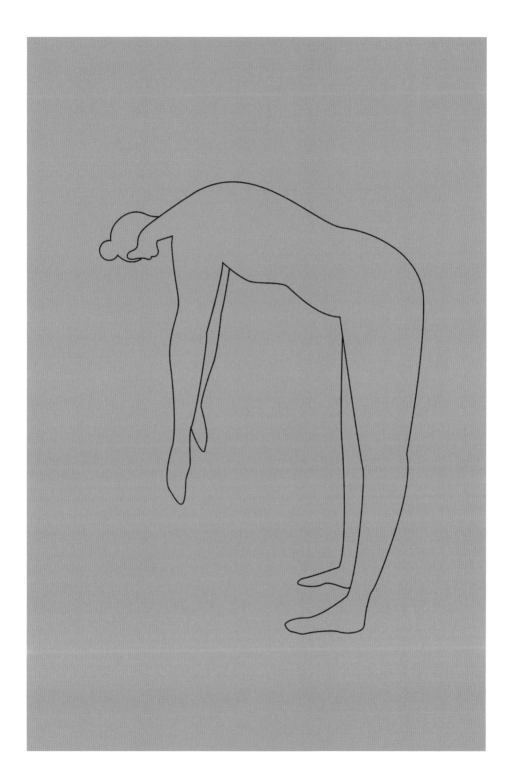

LISTEN, FEEL, REACT

When first performing a stretch, you get your body into a position and that's really what a stretch is – a position of the body. But what's next once you get into position? Do you just stay there and hope the time goes quickly?

The next thing is to feel the stretch: Does it feel nice, horrible, correct? Is it painful or can you feel nothing at all? Be interested, not judgemental, and don't make a big deal out of it.

Stretching is all about listening to your body and reacting to what it's telling you. If it feels painful, you have to make a change. If the stretching feeling eases off, you need to move deeper into the stretch. However, you also have to be aware enough to know when to stop and back off, and also be smart enough not to come out of a stretch just because the allocated time is up.

You're the only one who can know how a stretch feels. No matter how much I've studied, coached or repeated any particular position, I can never truly know how that feels for *you*. Listening to your body is so important as this is what will help you progress and keep you safe.

RED FLAGS

Here are a few examples of feelings / sensations that might come up for you and I assure you they are common for many people.

In Elevated Pigeon (page 112) do you feel any pinching in the knee?
In Rotation Twist with Wall (page 62) do you feel pressure on your head?
In Extension on Sofa (page 68) do you feel nothing?
In the Wall Arch (page 72) do you feel back pain?

The action we take is what determines whether we find a way through and this is where the variants come in (page 32). We must listen to our body and adapt the exercise or simply move on and try a different one. Don't give up after a tiny bit of discomfort. Adjust your position and do what is needed to keep on progressing.

DOES IT FEEL NICE, HORRIBLE, CORRECT?

PAIN IS GOOD

I think we can all agree that when you hear a baby crying it's a pretty hard noise to ignore. Why is that? Well, it's designed to get you to pay attention. That's what the baby wants – your attention. They may be hungry, thirsty or scared, but they're just expressing themselves and really couldn't care less whether you are busy or have a deadline. They are going to let you know.

Now, when you compare that to pain it's actually very similar. When you feel pain it's your body's cry for attention. Again, it can be for all sorts of reasons, whether it's pain from touching something hot, stepping on some glass, or that neck ache you wake up with on a daily basis. Pain does not care how busy you are, it's going to express to you how it feels.

If a baby had a volume button and I told you to fix the crying by just turning it down, then you might think I'm some kind of lunatic. Surely, it's up to us to try to figure out what their needs are and try to help them.

And pain – is it OK to turn down the volume on that one? Pain is your body's cry for help. The very last thing you should try to do is to turn that volume down because when you do you're numbing it and not giving your body what it wants. Please don't numb your pain – your very clever and smart body is trying to get a message through to you. Pay attention.

Pain is a sensation, a strong one, a strong enough sensation to stop you right in your tracks. That's its purpose, if it wasn't, you'd just keep your hands on a hot stove and cause long-term harm to your body. When your body feels pain, it sends you a signal and it's that signal that promotes action.

You could say that pain is the biggest motivation for action. Action begins from pain. If pain could speak it would say 'Do something!', so why do we have such a bad relationship with it? Why are we running around in circles trying to get rid of it?

So, what am I saying here? I am saying that whenever somebody tells me that they are experiencing pain I think 'phew'. I feel happy that their body is responding and forcing them to take action. And this is the same for me too. If I slack on my training or spend too much time sitting or writing, I expect to be in pain! If I'm not, I'm a little disappointed that my body isn't on the ball enough to give me a kick up the arse.

The number one motivator for a person to start any form of movement practice is their own body giving them that kick, and that kick is pain. One of the main reasons that you might be reading this book is because pain has brought you here. Pain was the trigger, the action step, the sensation that said 'enough', so please don't hate pain. I know it's not a pleasant sensation but if it was, it wouldn't do the same job. It has to be horrible, niggly, awful. It has to make you wince, cry and complain, that's its job.

I think pain is the action step to truly changing people's lives. I personally choose to never take painkillers or any type of drug that will dampen that sensation in my body. The pain signal is a message from your body and it's essential that you not only listen to that message but take it on board and take those action steps required. I'm all for medicine, but only when necessary.

'WHERE AM I SUPPOSED TO FEEL THE STRETCH?'

If I had a millimetre of flexibility for every time that I've heard this question, I'd be bendier than a contortionist. I'd say this is probably the most frequently asked question whenever I'm coaching, and I really want to address it in an in-depth way. You see, the question implies that a stretch is designed for a specific area of the body, which it is, as if everybody is tight in the same places. The problem is, they are not.

If I gave the same stretch to a group of five-year-olds, they'd be a lot more likely to feel it in the same place than if I gave that same stretch to a group of 40-year-olds. The reason for this is that life has happened (page 19). If we take three people as an example and one goes running occasionally, one doesn't exercise at all and the other does weights at the gym and all three have been doing this for a decade, then their bodies are going to be different in so many ways.

Imagine I'm in a room coaching a group of 20 people and I ask them all to do a forward fold and touch their toes. Do you think that all 20 of those people will be in exactly the same position? Absolutely not! When I'm coaching at events and I do this, I look around the room and see so many variations. Some people are barely past their thighs while others have their elbows on the floor – that is a huge range of flexibility.

So, can we say that the purpose of the exercise is the same? Yes, it's a forward fold. But can we say that all 20 people will feel the stretch in the same place? No way. Even if I make sure all their feet are facing forwards and all their knees are straight, I will still get feedback that points to different areas of the body. The feedback is real, it's what the person is feeling.

But surely, no matter where they are within that stretch, they are still stretching the same muscles? NO, they are not stretching the same muscles, they are stretching the same position, which is probably the hardest concept for people to grasp. The purpose is not to stretch muscles but to improve a position. The forward fold is the position and there are hundreds of muscles at work within that position. Calves, numerous hamstrings, butt, back, neck... plus all the other tendons, ligaments, joints and tissue surrounding and layering those areas.

It's not possible that all of these people are stretching the exact same muscles when it's obvious they are all in very different variations of the same position and are all giving very different feedback. They are not stretching the same muscles and nor should they be – they are all trying to improve this specific position.

As they improve upon that position, the consequences will be different muscles stretching for each of them; essentially whichever area is the most restricted.

There are hundreds of muscles in the body. It would be completely unrealistic and also impossible to work our way around the body trying to stretch each individual muscle separately, because to look at the body from this perspective is like trying to view the body as a collection of separate and individual muscles that don't interact with each other.

Every movement you make with your body takes millions of minuscule movements to make it happen. Every part of the body is connected to the next and you cannot isolate and stretch a single part of the body without affecting another part. The body is a unit of billions of moving parts and, when we put them together, it becomes a whole.

If you asked me how many muscles the body has, I would simply reply, 'One'. This is not only a much simpler idea but, based on the notion that all parts affect each other, viewing it as a whole is a much smarter and easier concept to grasp.

So today, let go of the idea of stretching individual muscles. We stretch a position and where you feel the stretch within that position is where you feel the stretch. In other words, you create a position and what comes up for you within that movement is perfect for you and is exactly what your body needs at that given moment.

THE PATH OF LEAST RESISTANCE

The path of least resistance describes how we subconsciously use our bodies in whichever way requires the least effort. Whether it's putting on your clothes in the morning, sending a text on your phone or having a shower. Every time you perform these tasks you will do so in a very similar way without thinking about it. These movements are your path of least resistance – this is where your body loves to be and also where it has learned to be because it's the easiest way to get the movement done. However, the more you repeat these movements, the more the message is reinforced that this is the way to do the task. Notice when you're sitting cross-legged, it's always the same leg in front – that's the path of least resistance at play.

When it comes to exercising, I have a very technical term for this – it's called 'cheating'. For years, it's been my job to watch myself and others try to cheat out of exercises and usually this is not on purpose but a subconscious choice. We think we are going into a specific position but, in reality, the body has just gone around the bit that needs our attention the most. Why would it do that? Well, it's like our comfort zone – why is it easier to go into a YouTube hole than to write a physics essay? One is effortless, one requires effort. The brain likes the first option because it's short term, whereas we know the second will feel more rewarding, perhaps not at the time, but later.

We are hardwired to want instant gratification. Right now, my brain does not want to write this book – if I stop writing now and go on social media, that will equal instant gratification. I will get a quick reward, followed by the need for more reward. However, if I persist, I will get a huge, much more satisfying and tangible reward further down the line. You might want to stop reading this book in order to get a hit of instant gratification elsewhere, but if you stay with me and take the time to read and understand the theory behind this book, you're going to have such an advantage when it comes to implementing your daily movements, and the huge long-term rewards they will bring.

MOBILITY VS FLEXIBILITY

Sometimes, these two words are used interchangeably when really they mean very different things. Instead of explaining the difference, I'm going to get you to *feel* the difference, using this simple exercise.

Sit on the floor with your legs out in front of you, now clasp your hands together underneath one of your thighs and pick up your leg so your foot is no longer touching the ground.

Now that you have the leg suspended, try to pull your thigh as close as you can to your chest. Depending on your flexibility, you may be able to do this with your leg straight. If you can, keep the leg straight, if not, keep a slight bend in the knee.

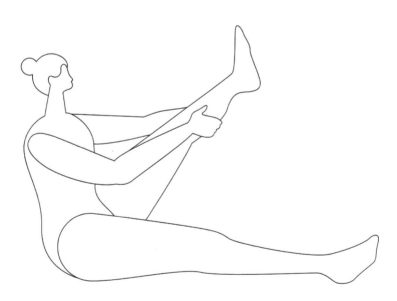

The point where you can bring the leg to shows your flexibility and your maximum range of motion within this specific position. To test your mobility, you need to hold the leg at the same height without any help from your hands, except there's a catch. Try the exercise and experience it for yourself before reading on to find out what that problem is.

Did you find the problem? You have probably just realized that you can't achieve the same height without assistance. This is because, when you let go, you are no longer testing for flexibility, but for mobility – mobility is the range you can actually use and reach with no assistance. There's little point in having all this range of motion if you can't actually use it.

So, to clarify: the seven movements in this book focus on improving both your mobility and flexibility, so sometimes you will feel a stretching sensation and other times a strengthening sensation. It's equally important to train both. If you're thinking, 'hang on a minute, this book is called *Stretch* and I'm feeling a lot of effort', that's OK. You're training your mobility, which will also increase your flexibility.

Flexibility = your maximum range of motion when the muscles are relaxed (assisted)

Mobility = your maximum range of motion using those muscles within a specific position (unassisted)

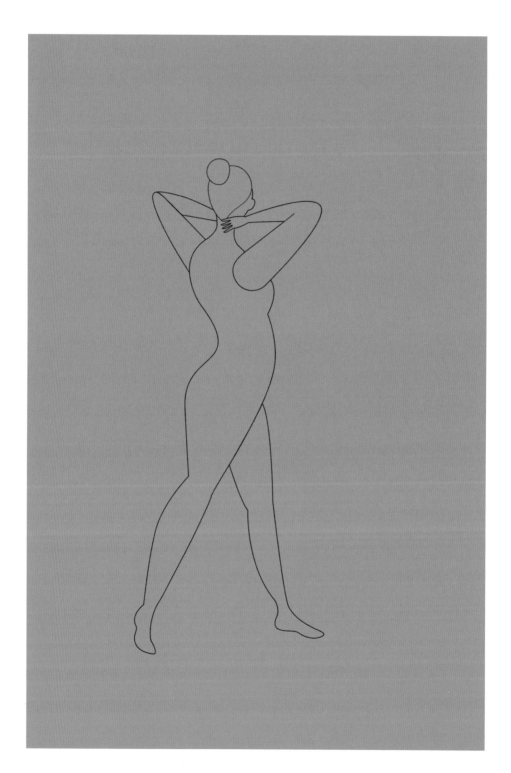

A NOTE ON SHOULDER PAIN

If your shoulders are not functioning as they should, it can be a real issue. However, what can be even more problematic is if, when you're trying to get them moving back to how they should, you experience pain, pinching or discomfort, which can make you question the point of stretching at all. What I say is, you can't just ignore your body for decades and then suddenly go back to it and expect it to be totally fine.

When it comes to the body, time doesn't heal and ignorance just buries the pain for a later date. Naturally, we all want to get to the point where we can easily sink into a nice stretch without any discomfort and you will get there, but this will take repetition. You need to be patient, consistent and never give up. The great thing is that your journey to this point has already begun.

There is no way I could write a book about the most essential stretches and not mention hanging (see page 102). One of the ways I've regained my shoulder health and flexibility is through regular hanging. Hanging is a primitive movement that comes naturally to us and does wonders for our shoulder health.

Dr John Kirsch, an orthopedic surgeon with over 30 years' experience, recommends in his book *Shoulder Pain?* that we spend time hanging each day. You will find alternatives to hanging on pages 92 and 100, but to experience the real thing I suggest any of the following:

+ Finding a safe place outside you can hang from, such as a playground or outdoor gym (I recommend the app Calisthenics Parks for this)

+ Purchasing something you can hang from. A door frame bar or an aluminium bar.

THE SEVEN ESSENTIAL STRETCHES

THE PROGRAMME

You'll notice I write on each exercise: 'Do the movement for your chosen time'. But how long is that and what am I doing when I'm in the stretch?

HOW TO STRETCH

> You have two options that are equally powerful, so it is really down to personal preference.

OPTION 1: STATIC

Static means still but I don't mean you to be frozen solid with no option of movement. With any stretch, you first need to find where the stretch is for you. That requires a little bit of feeling around and making sure that you don't feel pain – the type of pain that indicates there is something not quite right (see Red Flags on page 36). Imagine feeling your way around a room at night with the light switched off – you really need to use all your attention to feel where everything is. That is exactly what you want to be like when stretching.

If you're doing the static option in the stretch, you want to be as still as possible but always looking to increase the stretch. For example, the position that you start in should be different from the one that you end up in. Set up the position, feel that the stretch is right for you, then gradually increase the stretch over a 2-minute period, breathing outwards as you get deeper into the stretch.

OPTION 2: MOVING

Moving does not mean fidgeting; your body is going to do everything in its power to avoid the stretch and feel the least stretch possible. When you move in the stretch, you want to move slowly between a light sense of stretch and an increased sense of stretch. Let me give an example.

1	2	3	4	5	6	7	8	9	10

If number one represents a super light feeling of stretch and number ten represents the strongest stretch possible, you want to move slowly between the lower numbers and the higher numbers but pause for a few seconds at the most intense part. Try to avoid holding your breath as then the body won't relax – really focus on the out breath at the most intense point.

HOW LONG TO STRETCH FOR

Each stretch should be performed according to your chosen level.

Follow the programme above. You are working your way up to Level 6. Start at

LEVEL 1 = 1 MINUTE PER EXERCISE. 1 ROUND. TOTAL = 7 MINUTES
(less than 1 per cent of your day – THE BARE MINIMUM)

LEVEL 2 = 2 MINUTES PER EXERCISE. 1 ROUND. TOTAL = 14 MINUTES
(less than 2 per cent of your day)

LEVEL 3 = 3 MINUTES PER EXERCISE. 1 ROUND. TOTAL = 21 MINUTES
(less than 2.5 per cent of your day)

LEVEL 4 = 2 MINUTES PER EXERCISE X 2 ROUNDS. TOTAL = 28 MINUTES
(less then 3 per cent of your day)

LEVEL 5 = 2 MINUTES PER EXERCISE X 3 ROUNDS. TOTAL = 42 MINUTES
(less than 5 per cent of your day)

LEVEL 6 = 3 MINUTES PER EXERCISE X 3 ROUNDS. TOTAL = 1 HOUR, 3 MINUTES
(less then 7 per cent of your day)

Level 1. Once you manage to do Level 1 for 7 days in a row, move to Level 2. Keep moving up the levels until you reach Level 6. Consistency wins the day.

HOW TO FIT THE EXERCISES INTO YOUR EVERYDAY LIFE

Each exercise has three variations. All you need is seven movements; the rest are options for increasing intensity. To make it super easy for you to get started, we've not only created a programme for the first week but we have also made a little memo card for you. It's the same size as an ID or credit card, so it sits perfectly inside your wallet, or you can take a picture of it for your phone.

My seven movements for today are:

	EXERCISE	TIME
☐	WALL PYRAMID (FLEXION)	_____
☐	EXTENSION ON A SOFA / TABLE (EXTENSION)	_____
☐	BROOMSTICK TWIST (ROTATION)	_____
☐	WALL SLIDES (LATERAL FLEXION)	_____
☐	REVERSE SHOULDER STRETCH (SHOULDERS)	_____
☐	LAZY WALL STRETCH (HIPS)	_____
☐	FEET IN FRONT (BALANCE)	_____

I suggest using this programme for the first week, no matter your level and even if you don't find it very challenging at all. The first aim is consistency and forming a habit. Once your week is over, you can then start to try the more challenging variations of the essential seven.

For example, you can make the rotations more advanced or perhaps just make the balance harder. The exercises have really been designed so that, no matter what level you are at, you can design your own programme. On the next page, you will find a sample timetable where you can create your own programme as there are lots of possibilities for mixing it up and making your movements unique to you.

	1	2	3	4	5	6	7
MONDAY	MOVE	MOVE	MOVE	MOVE	MOVE	MOVE	MOVE
TUESDAY	MOVE	MOVE	MOVE	MOVE	MOVE	MOVE	MOVE
WEDNESDAY	MOVE	MOVE	MOVE	MOVE	MOVE	MOVE	MOVE
THURSDAY	MOVE	MOVE	MOVE	MOVE	MOVE	MOVE	MOVE
FRIDAY	MOVE	MOVE	MOVE	MOVE	MOVE	MOVE	MOVE
SATURDAY	MOVE	MOVE	MOVE	MOVE	MOVE	MOVE	MOVE
SUNDAY	MOVE	MOVE	MOVE	MOVE	MOVE	MOVE	MOVE

THERE ARE TWO MAIN WAYS YOU CAN GET THE MOVEMENTS IN THROUGHOUT THE DAY:

A. Do them all in one go.

B. Spread them throughout the day. When we took this to an Instagram poll, 75 per cent of people said they would rather do all the movements in one go. Personally, I much prefer to tick them off and get on with my day but, if you prefer to spread them throughout the day, here's how that might look:

1.	**MORNING: BALANCE**
2.	**MID-MORNING: SPINE ROTATION**
3.	**MIDDAY: HIPS**
4.	**MID-AFTERNOON: SHOULDERS**
5.	**LATE AFTERNOON: SPINE LATERAL FLEXION**
6.	**EVENING: SPINE EXTENSION**
7.	**LATE EVENING: SPINE FLEXION**

Head to www.roger.coach, where we have digital cards for you to create your programme on and remember, every day it's the same: **4 x spine, hips, shoulders and balance.**

WHAT YOU'LL NEED

EQUIPMENT

Most of these exercises can be performed without any equipment at all but you may find the following pieces useful for regular practice. I really don't mind where you get them, but I promise they will be worth it and you'll hopefully use them thousands of times.

ESSENTIAL EQUIPMENT:

+ Mat (especially if you have wooden floors)
+ A couple of yoga blocks (blocks not bricks)
+ Yoga belt
+ A broomstick (without the head)
+ Exercise loop bands

HERE ARE SOME FREE ALTERNATIVES YOU MIGHT ALREADY HAVE AT HOME:

+ Books instead of yoga blocks.
+ Regular belt or dressing gown cord instead of yoga belt

BONUS

+ Something to hang from (a door bar or some kind of frame)

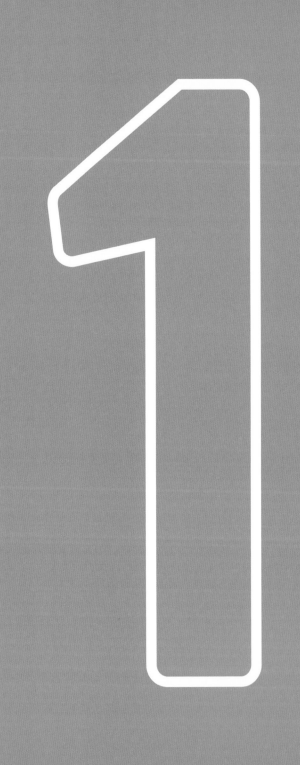

SPINE
ROTATION

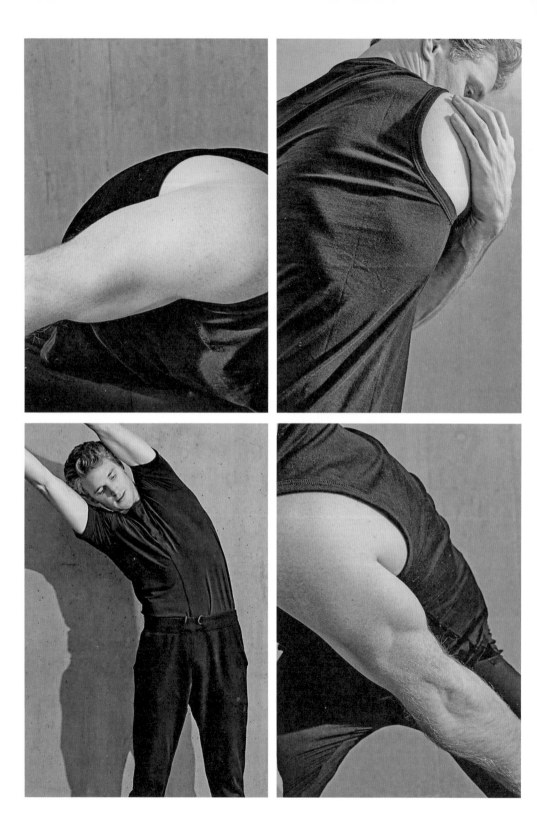

SPINE ROTATION

You are as old as your spine, so in this section we will be looking at one of the fundamental movements of the human body: rotation. Like all movements, if we don't use them, we lose them! So, it's essential to keep your spine in check and teach it to perform the motions it must do regularly.

You'll notice, when we are doing rotational exercises, that we do them sitting on the floor. When standing, too much rotation can end up occurring through the knees or hips, whereas sitting encourages or rather forces rotation through the trunk.

Our sedentary culture means that our back is often in a flexed position for far too long and our upper back, where the majority of our rotation should come from, has been in a frozen position for many years. (You'll see the same story when it comes to Extension.) This can also be the case if you have been focused on specific sports that don't use rotation or concentrated more on weight loss/gain or muscle gain.

For a whole variety of reasons, it's very easy for simple spinal rotation to be left on the back burner and so, as one of the most neglected ranges of motion, I will be reintroducing it as one of your essential seven daily stretches.

ROTATION 1: BROOMSTICK TWIST

For this first rotation exercise, you'll need a stick. Hopefully, you can find a broomstick in the kitchen that will do the trick. Alternatively, holding a block or book in your hands will work just fine.

Note: Due to weight distribution, I suggest taking the head off the broom before using it for this exercise.

HOW TO DO IT...

Sit on the floor in a cross-legged position. If you cannot sit fully upright in this position, place a block or two under your butt. Sitting rather than standing when doing this exercise stops the movement coming from the hips so you get more movement through your torso and spine.

Next, pick up the stick and hold it horizontally around shoulder height. If you feel any pain or pinching at this point, lower the stick accordingly.

Now, holding the body upright, rotate from the centre slowly to the left and back again for your chosen time, pausing for a few seconds once you reach your maximum rotation and then repeating the movement on the opposite side for the same time. Keep your hips glued to the floor and follow the centre of the stick with your head, ensuring that the movement is coming through the upper body and the spine.

Once you have completed the rotation for your chosen time, repeat the stretch on the other side of your body.

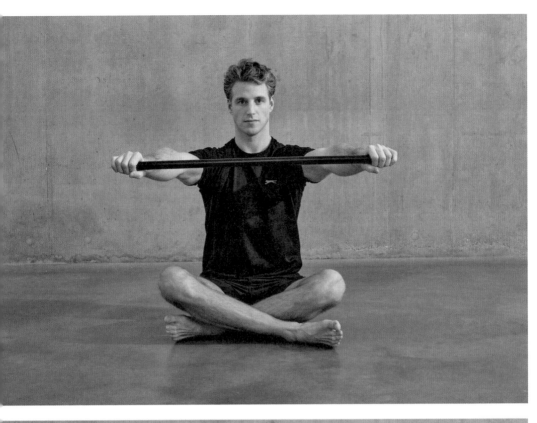

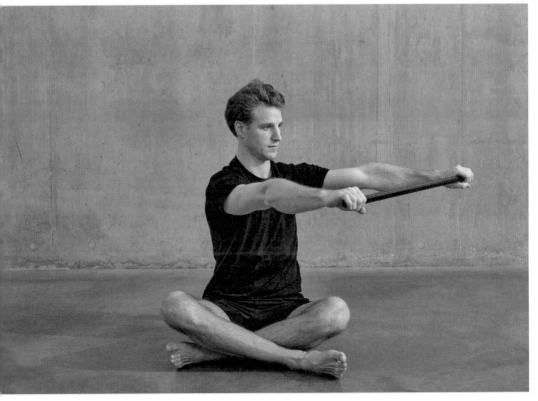

ROTATION 2: SOFA TWIST

The Sofa Twist is a way to get rotation in your spine while having minimal pressure on your head and neck. You do need to think about the height of your sofa here and make any adjustments necessary to adapt this exercise to suit your needs.

The Sofa Twist is a toned-down variation of a full gymnastic exercise where the head is on the floor. You are more than welcome to try the head-on-the-floor variation (please find this on the following page) but take care to ensure you are rotating from the middle of the spine and not just in the hips and neck. The rule of thumb is this: the lower the surface you are working on with the rested shoulder, the more advanced the exercise becomes. Start with the height of a sofa and work your way towards the floor using blocks.

HOW TO DO IT...

Start kneeling on the floor in front of a sofa or similar, with your knees about hip-width apart. Reach your left arm underneath your body to the left, resting the outside of your left shoulder on the surface and creating a twist with the upper body.

Once in the position, rest your head on the sofa / surface and place your right palm on top of your left. From here, moving slowly, raise the right hand to stretch the arm up to the ceiling and then hold for your chosen time, focusing on squeezing your right shoulder blade back and down and turning your chest towards the ceiling.

If holding your arm up in the air is tiring at first, a good option is to place your free hand behind your back, towards your opposite pocket. So, if you are lying on your left shoulder, you should take the back of your right hand to the left hip.

When you are in the stretch, push the right hip backwards to keep your hips square – this will ensure the rotation is coming from the spine only. You are more likely to feel this stretch when you come out of it, so don't be overly concerned if you don't really feel much of a stretch at the time of doing it.

Repeat on the opposite side. Test your rotation using the Broomstick Twist on page 58 in between rotations to see if you notice an improvement.

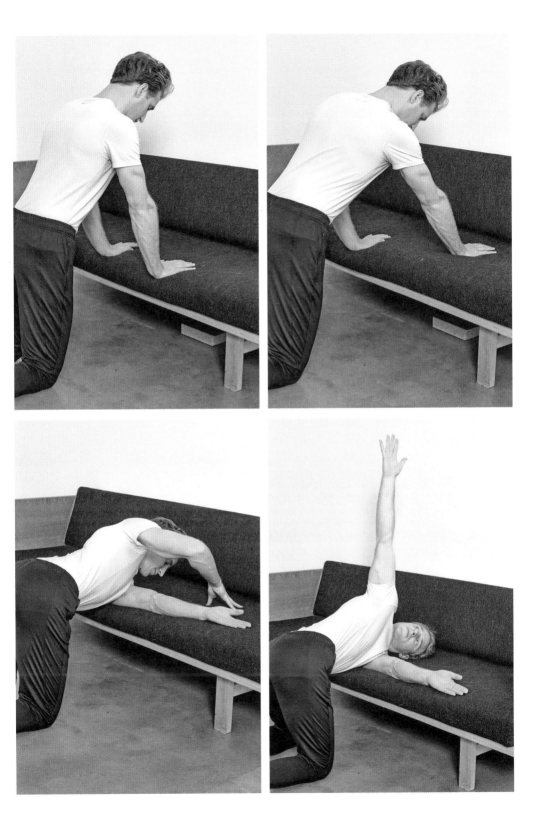

ROTATION 3: ROTATION TWIST WITH WALL

This is a deeper variation of the Sofa Twist (page 60). If you feel like there is pressure on the neck or the stretch is too intense for you, revert back to the Sofa Twist or place blocks underneath the shoulder on the floor. This exercise can build up to quite an extreme twist, especially when using the wall, which is what your body needs, but you need to take time to build up to it.

If this exercise feels like a big step, an option to make it easier is to place a block or two between your shoulder and the floor as this will reduce the angle to the floor.

HOW TO DO IT...

Start on all fours, facing the wall, with your head almost touching the wall. Drop the left arm and place the outside of your left shoulder on the floor, aiming to keep your hips directly above your knees.

Next, reach your right hand above your head and on to the wall – this creates an extra pull to rotate the spine open. As you lift the hand, make sure that your hips don't twist out of line. This is the biggest mistake. All of the twist should be coming from the torso so check the hips are directly above the knees.

+ look up towards the ceiling (careful on the neck)
+ keep the hips square
+ extend the right arm up the wall

To increase the stretch, walk your right hand further down the wall, away from your head. Repeat on the opposite side, testing your rotation in between using the Broomstick Twist on page 58.

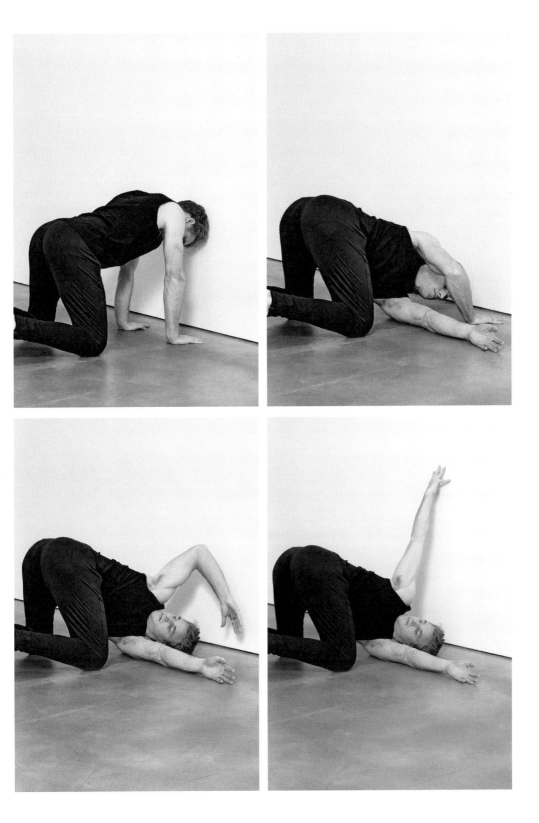

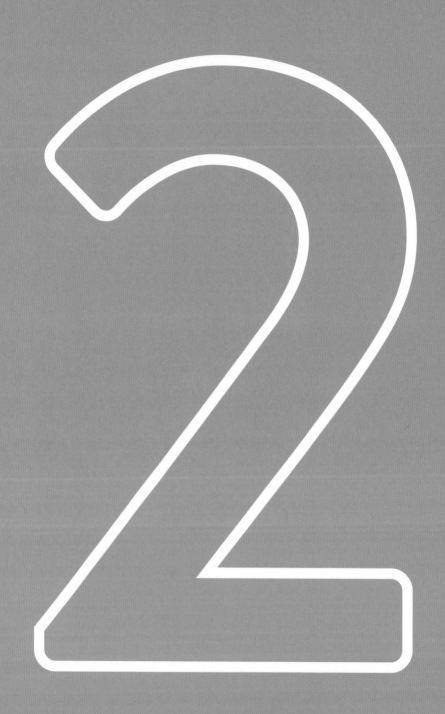

SPINE EXTENSION

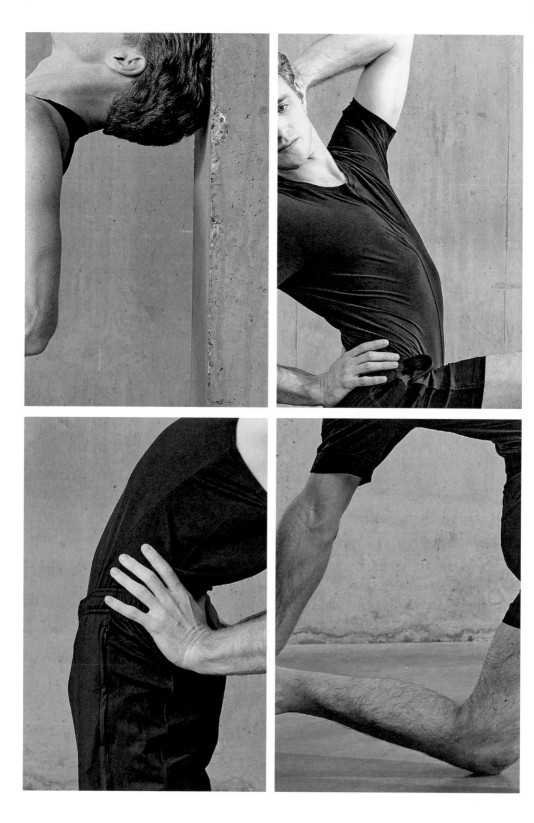

SPINE EXTENSION

Before diving into extension, let's talk a little bit about back pain, as it's likely to come up here. It is common for a lot of people to have experienced pain in the lower back. Perhaps you are currently experiencing it. If so, I'm glad you're here with me as we focus on this particular area and get you some relief through increased movement.

The way we currently live our lives – sitting too much and working on laptops – means that our backs are in a flexed position for far too long. Extension of the spine is the opposite of flexion. Point your rib cage to the sky or the ceiling right now – lift it up. Well done, you just gave your spine some extension.

Ideally, when extending your spine, you want to get the majority of that movement from your upper back or thoracic spine. It's safer to extend the spine here as this part of the spine has the rib cage attached. However, if this part of the spine has essentially become welded together through lack of use, you start to generate extension from the lower back, which doesn't have the same support from the rib cage. This can cause lower back pain, which can lead to you wanting to avoid extension entirely.

Avoiding the movement altogether isn't the answer, as this doesn't fix the fact that your spine needs to extend! In this book I will be reintroducing extension of the spine in a safe way to reopen your upper back while avoiding any tension in the lower back. It's important to listen to your body here. Your body will certainly let you know if you're going down the wrong route. Choose any one of the next three exercises and find something doable to get you started.

EXTENSION 1: EXTENSION ON SOFA / TABLE

I love this exercise; not only is it simple to perform, it's one of the safest exercises you can do and it's actually one of the 'nicer' stretches. The sensation of the stretch is very calm, and I would definitely say it's more of a relaxing stretch than most, so it's ideal to do just before bed or to help you relax in the evening. That said, it doesn't mean it's not as beneficial as any of the other stretches. You'll certainly feel this but, more than likely, it'll be once you come out of the stretch.

HOW TO DO IT...

Slouch down your sofa to the front edge, keeping your upper back and shoulders in contact with the cushions and your feet planted on the floor, hip-width apart. When starting this exercise, you want a soft surface, although it's completely fine to use a harder one. It's more a matter of comfort than results.

Next, push your pelvis down towards the floor. You are trying to get your pelvis as close as you can to the floor but without touching. If you can reach the floor, you need a higher surface and I suggest using the arm or back of the sofa, or even a small table with a couple of soft blocks or a mat on for comfort. Your pelvis should be suspended above the floor.

As you push your pelvis down towards the floor, you want to keep your shoulders in contact with the surface you're using, whether that is a sofa or a table. This will create some supported extension for your spine. In the image, you can see I am holding the back of my head in my hands. You can also try resting your head on the surface you are using but keep focusing on pushing the pelvis down.

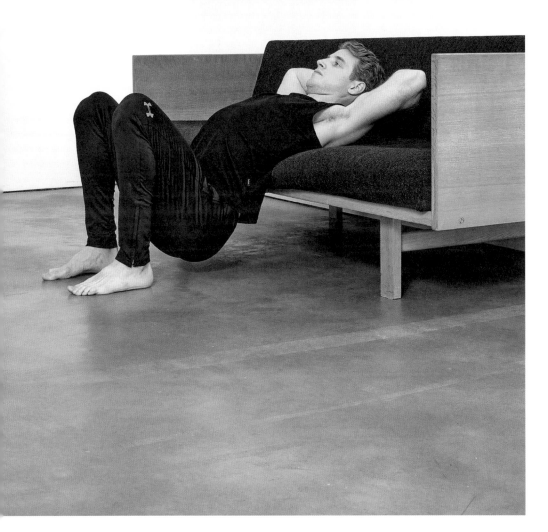

EXTENSION 2: CROSS-BODY STRETCH

This stretch creates extension in the spine but also includes a little bit of rotation. If there is tightness in the front of your body, you will also feel stretch in your thighs, hip flexors, sides and potentially even your stomach. All or any of these are great.

You really want to focus on opening up the front of the body here, especially if you're spending a lot of time sitting. Performing this stretch in a kneeling position protects the lower back from any excess movement, creating more movement in the upper back and hips. You can also add a modification: If you stand in front of a sofa, instead of reaching for your back heel, place your hand on the sofa instead, or place a couple of blocks next to your back heel to bring the floor closer to you. Work towards placing your hand on your foot and eventually the floor.

HOW TO DO IT...

Start in a lunge position with your right foot forwards and left knee on the floor. Feel free to pad up or put a mat underneath your knee to stop it digging into the floor. Place your left hand behind your head for support and your right arm on the back of your right hip.

You may already feel a decent stretch here – if so, remain here. However, there are a few options to move further. Either reach back and place your right hand on a sofa / table or place a couple of blocks next to your left heel and work towards putting your right hand there, backing off at any point should you feel any pinching or pain. Once you have got your hand in contact with the surface you are reaching back to, push your hips forward to increase the stretch. Once held for the chosen time, repeat on the opposite side.

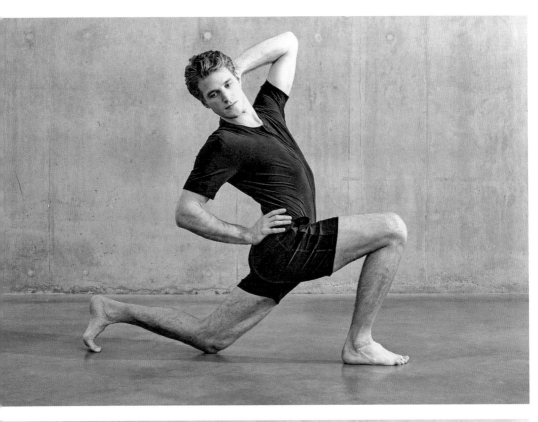

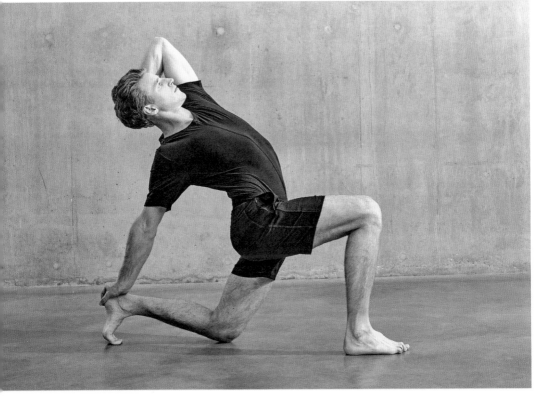

EXTENSION 3: WALL ARCH

The final progression in the extension stretches is the Wall Arch. This is a really good exercise for a slouchy or forward head posture, creating some decent extension in the spine. If you feel any neck pain when doing this exercise, place your hands on the back of your neck. As you progress, you'll be able to do it without using the wall for support.

HOW TO DO IT...

First, find a wall and, looking up, choose a spot on the ceiling that you don't mind staring at for a while. This exercise can feel surprisingly challenging and not just the movement itself but also from the heart rate rising and the breathing.

Next, kneel directly underneath your mark with your back to the wall. I have my toes flipped but, if you prefer, you can also try this with your feet the other way around so you are on the front of your feet. (Just preference). Place your hands at the sides of your lower back and then take the back of your head to the wall, looking up at your spot on the ceiling.

When in the stretch, focus on squeezing the shoulder blades back and down and facing your chest upwards towards the ceiling, as demonstrated in the photo. As with any exercise, back off if you feel any pain. Also, feel free at first to place a block or two or a couple of cushions between your head and the wall and even just have the hands relaxed down by your sides. This will take pressure off the back and build up the exercise slowly for you.

The important thing in the stretch is also to focus on squeezing your butt muscles and pushing your hips forwards. This will start to increase the arch and the head will move lower down the wall, thereby increasing the amount of extension in the spine.

Options to increase intensity: Take the knees further from the wall / remove the wall altogether.

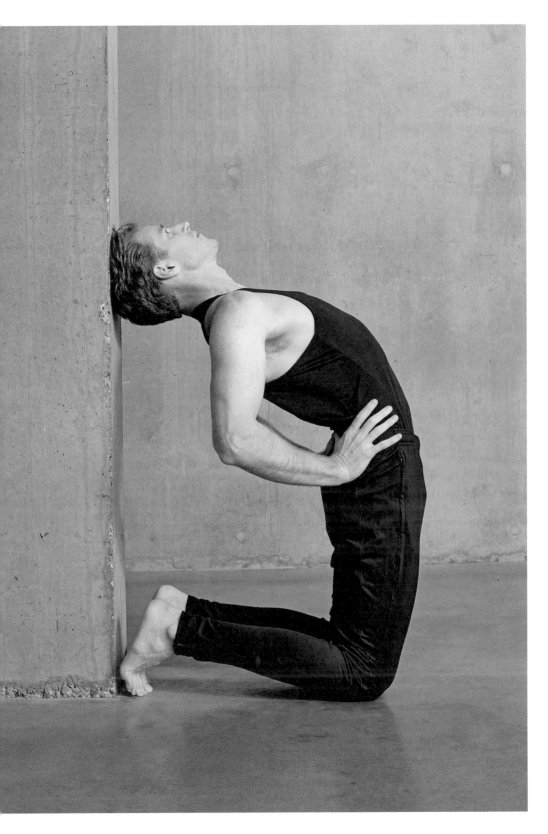

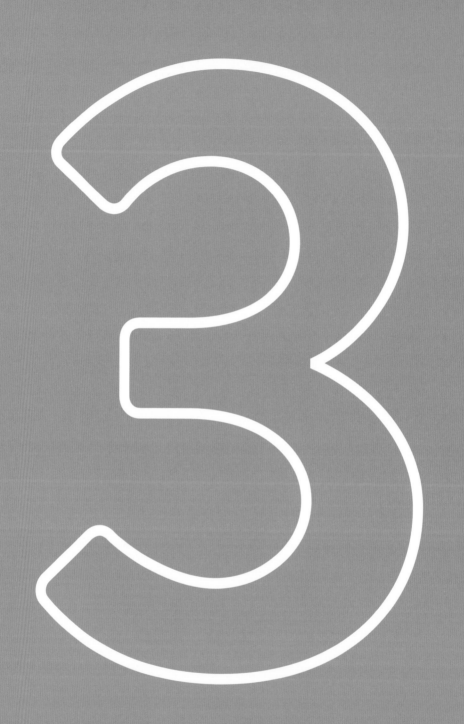

SPINE
FLEXION

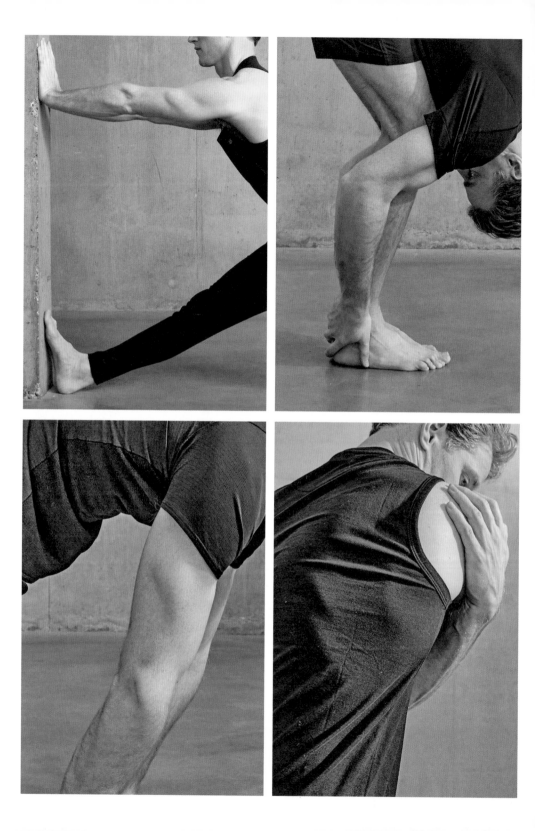

SPINE FLEXION

Touching your toes is probably the most well-known and obvious stretch. Your spine flexes when you reach down to touch your toes or pick something up off the floor. However, it's only stretching in one direction and we want to open up the body in ALL directions.

Throughout life, we are constantly fighting gravity. When standing bolt upright, gravity's force is straight down on top of our heads, but when we start to tilt our heads down or over-flex, gravity starts to hit the back of our heads or necks, causing extreme flexion, which many of us will see occurring in our parents or grandparents as they age. In this book, we will be using flexion to lengthen the body and help separate the vertebrae and stop them compressing into each other.

It is also important to say that it is completely fine to round your spine. We often have the idea that we should always have a perfectly straight spine. Yes, you want an elongated spine but flexing the spine is a great way to start that. Over time, as you lengthen all the muscles and tissue around the spine and the legs, the spine will become flatter or longer. But you need to start somewhere and flexing the spine will start that journey perfectly for you. Flexing the spine isn't wrong, it's just a consequence of tightness elsewhere in the body. In fact, when bending down to touch your toes, the more your spine is rounding, the tighter your legs are. As you resolve any tightness in the legs by consistently stretching them in numerous directions, the spine will become flatter / straighter as a result.

SPINE FLEXION 1: WALL PYRAMID

The mirror test
Before doing this exercise for the first time, give this mirror test a try.

Stand side-on in front of a mirror and fold down to try and touch your toes. Now look at your hips – are they behind your heels or above them? The goal, over time, is to get the hips above the heels. Here is where the wall will come in handy. You can use the wall to press your bodyweight forwards. Make sure you keep some weight in your heels though – don't go so far that you feel like you are going to fall over.

When you go into a forward fold, you can opt to use gravity to hang down and stretch the body or you can use a little bit of external resistance – in this case, a wall.

Using the wall not only gives you a little bit of extra pressure but also helps you to get the weight forward.

HOW TO DO IT...
Grab yourself a chair or small table and place it in front of you before setting up this stretch. As you improve you can use blocks, like I am demonstrating in the image. Stand flush against a wall with your legs a little wider than hip-width apart. There should be two points of contact with the wall: your heels and your butt.

Now, keeping the legs straight and both the heels and butt in contact with the wall, support yourself with your chosen object. Remember to keep the legs completely straight (no bending the knees here). You can be as high up as you need to be to make this work (hence the chair option). The wider the legs, the easier the exercise, so have the feet as wide as you need to at first.

As you progress, you can start bringing the feet closer together, dropping down through various block heights and eventually removing the object altogether.

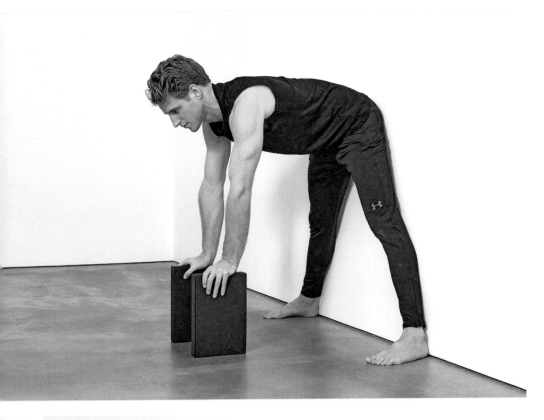

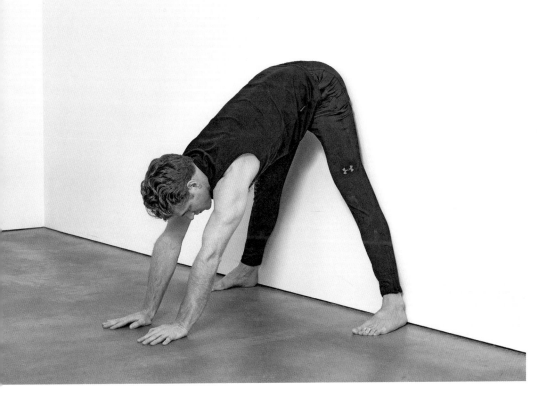

SPINE FLEXION 2: ANKLE GRAB

The objective here is for your chest to touch your thighs and I would definitely say this is more of a mobility than flexibility exercise (see Flexibility vs Mobility, page 42). Here, you will be using your upper body strength to compress the body in two. Over time, you won't need as much strength in the upper body or legs to do this.

Good news – you can bend the knees as much as you wish in this exercise. You are working on folding but, in this particular exercise, it's more important to get the chest compressed onto the thighs – the legs will straighten as you improve.

HOW TO DO IT...

Start standing with your feet together (although to begin with, hip-width apart isn't an issue). Fold forwards, bending your knees as much as you need in order to be able to place your chest firmly on your thighs. You want to be able to feel a point of contact between the chest and your thighs. Once that gap is closed as much as possible, relax the head and grab your ankles. If you can't reach the ankles at first, you can grab any point on the back of your legs.

As you pull, bend your arms and pull your upper body towards your lower body. In terms of the legs, focus on pushing the butt up but not so much that the upper body and lower body separate. Over time, you will be able to get the legs straighter. This can feel like quite an intense exercise on the thighs as you are using compression. It is a great exercise for stretching the back and also strengthening the legs. You'll get better each time you do it.

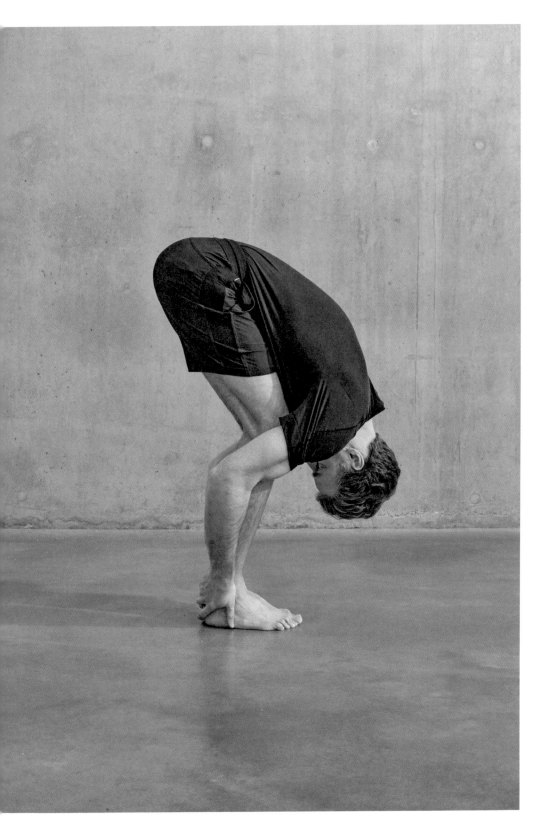

SPINE FLEXION 3: HEEL TO THE WALL

The great thing about this stretch is that it's easy to keep your back straight and you can also use the wall for support. If at first you can't reach the wall, a block will come in handy, as shown. If you find your heel or knee digging into the floor, use mats and blocks to resolve this. The blocks are really there to support you so that you can focus fully on the stretch. In all stretches we look for a sensation of stretch in the muscles and not a digging into the ground with the joints or bones. Be comfortable in your set-up so you can be focused on your stretch!

HOW TO DO IT...

Start facing a wall with a block in hand, if needed, and set up a lunge position with your right leg forwards. Straighten your right leg and try to get the heel of the foot as tight as you can to the wall with the toes facing directly upwards. Don't be too concerned about a gap between the heel and the wall at first as this will close over time.

Working from the feet up, the front foot faces upwards with the front thigh engaged to keep the front leg straight. To get maximum stretch, push the hips back slightly, especially on the right side. Doing so will increase the stretch. See What is Stretching on pages 30–31 to understand why we need two forces in each stretch.

Place your fingertips or block on the wall to keep your body upright. Lift the rib cage and, over time, work the head closer towards the wall. Focus on keeping the back straight and tall throughout the stretch and then repeat on the opposite side.

Options to increase intensity: Work towards having the heel closer to the wall / taking the knee further back over time.

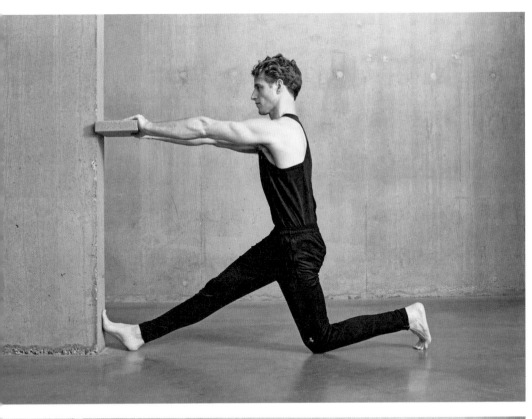

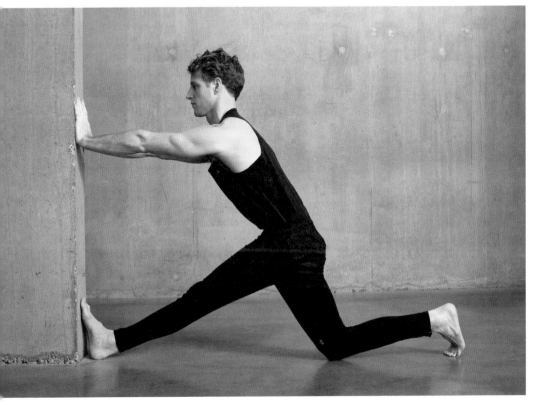

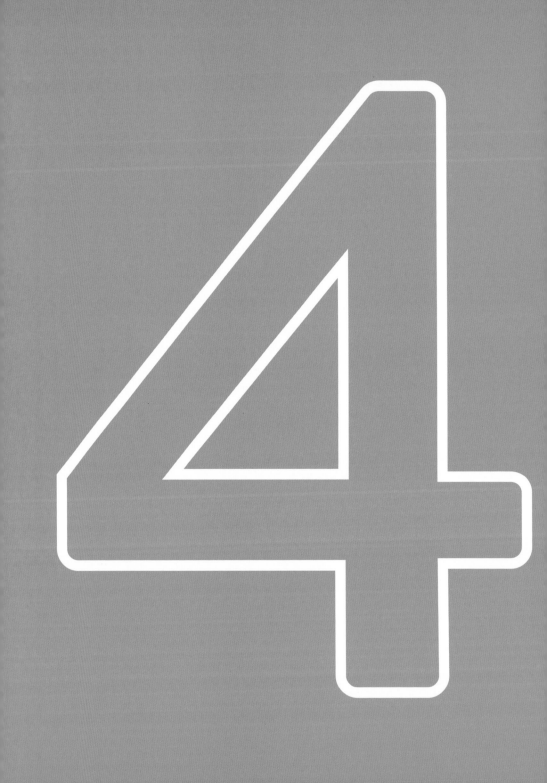

LATERAL
FLEXION

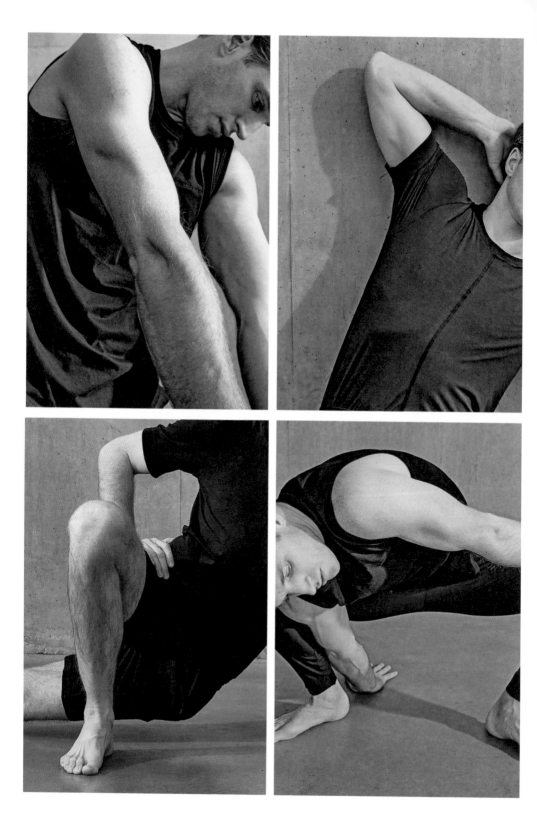

LATERAL FLEXION

Think of the tight or problem areas you would like to address, or about the reason you picked up this book. Was your inspiration to have flexible sides? Our first thought when it comes to flexibility is hamstrings, hips, shoulders or back but targeting the sides will impact all of these areas too.

When stretching our sides, the body tends to pull out of position and compensate by either pushing the hips forwards or backwards and tricking us into thinking that we're more flexible than we are in that area. We need to be aware of this or we're really missing out on what needs the most attention.

Stand up tall, and reach as far as you can down the outside of your leg towards your knee. You're now creating lateral flexion. You will notice that the first exercise in this chapter that uses lateral flexion is being done against a wall. This is to ensure that the movement is coming purely from the trunk of the body and you are not compensating with the hips.

Doing this really puts the focus on the sides of your body and will help you get used to what your body is 'avoiding', see more on the Path of Least Resistance on page 41. I will be reintroducing lateral flexion (side body stretching) as a standard daily movement to keep your body free from injuries and pain. In the following stretches, your objective is to 'find the stretch' or find the part of your body that needs your attention the most. The body is forever trying to trick us out of it. It's down to us to be fully aware of our body at all times and pay attention to the position of our body in these stretches.

LATERAL FLEXION 1: WALL SLIDES

In this exercise you will be using a wall to stretch the sides of your body. The wall will help to stop your body from rotating out of the stretch so you can keep an eye on the position of the body when in the stretch. There are a few variations of this exercise, so try the different options to see which is the best fit for you.

HOW TO DO IT...

Start sitting with your back against a wall. Make sure you can feel your back against the wall as you need to keep the focus there when you go into the side stretch. There will be two main contact points for your body on the wall: the sacrum (underneath your lower back), and your upper back. The objective is to keep these points in contact with the wall at all times as you move through the exercise.

You can see in the image I'm demonstrating this in a cross-legged position, but you could also have the soles of the feet together 'butterfly', or the legs straight, or one leg straight, one leg bent, whichever is comfortable. Once you have your set-up and the right points in contact, place your right hand behind your head and slide your left hand along the floor.

As you go into the stretch, make sure you keep the right buttock in contact with the ground. If this comes off the floor, you have gone too far. Slide as far as you can with your left hand and pause when you have reached your limit.

For added stretch, bring your right hand up and straighten your arm, reaching your right arm as far to the left as you can, as shown in the image. Hold or move slowly in and out of the stretch for your chosen time and then repeat on the opposite side.

Quick Tip: If, with the hand behind your head, you feel any pinching in the shoulder, you can find a more comfortable position for it; either down by your side or holding the arm out straight at shoulder height.

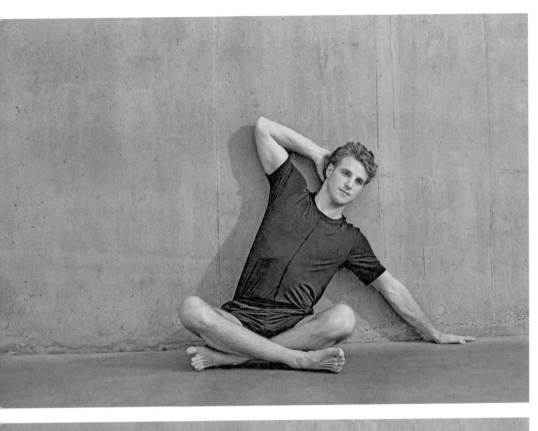

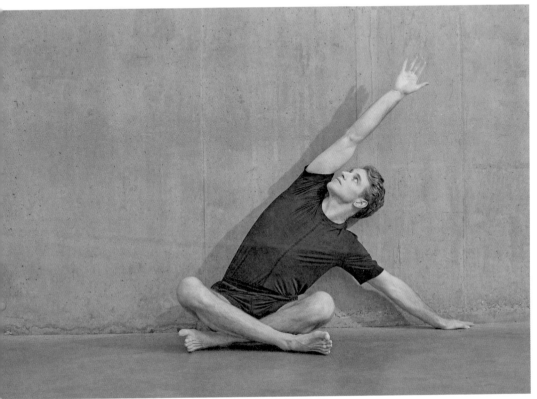

LATERAL FLEXION 2: SIDE BODY STRETCH

This side stretch may require a little bit of strength in the straight arm to hold you upright and, like many stretches, it requires exploration. I don't mean to sound too spiritual here, but stretches don't just happen to us, they need to be found / explored / played with. The words I'm using aren't important. What is important is that you know there are so many possibilities for this stretch.

Follow the steps below to perform this stretch:

1. Copy the image.
2. See if you feel something.
3. If you do, stay there.
4. If you don't, read the text below in case you have missed anything.
5. If you feel something, stay there.
6. If you don't feel anything, explore the position until you feel a stretch.
7. Repeat on the opposite side.

What do I mean by 'explore'? There are so many possible changes that you can make to a position, but it requires you to have an open mind. With this position, for example, the distance between the hand and the hip can change, the hip can push forwards or back, the bent leg foot position and knee positions can change – maybe the knee goes towards the floor and you roll on the ankle a bit. What about the outside of the straight leg – can you roll more onto the side?

Do you see the infinite possibilities available to 'create' stretches? There are always miniscule changes that you can make to change how the stretch works for you.

You might think, 'But I'm not a movement coach – how will I know if I am doing it right?' You will know when it feels right and you will also know when it doesn't feel right. This is the beauty of the body. It constantly gives us feedback on whether positions are right for us or not and we can react to that by making miniscule changes. However, if you get too caught up in the precise positioning of the stretch, then you're not really working with the body or paying attention to the feedback that it gives you.

Always remember this: the best movers on this planet are not coaches, therapists or teachers, and definitely not me. The best movers are toddlers. How often are they practising? All day long. Who are they being taught by? Themselves! The lesson to be learnt here is that we were moving our bodies before we were speaking. Try and get your head around that!

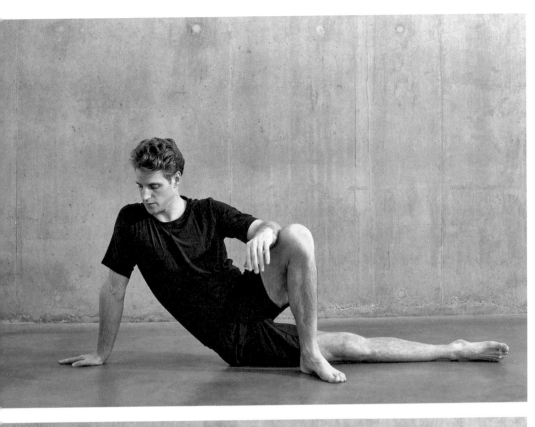

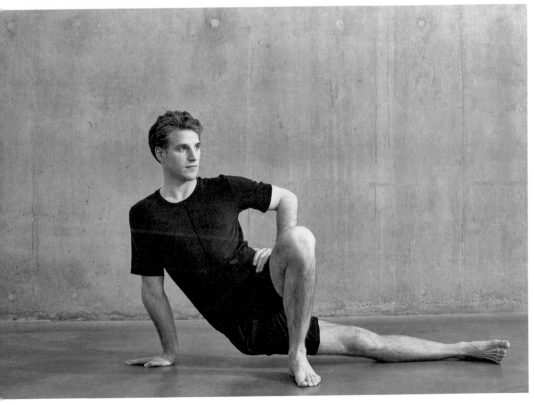

LATERAL FLEXION 3: DOOR FRAME STRETCH

For the third and final stretch in the side series, how could I not bring in the Door Frame Stretch? I have done this stretch thousands of times and I really like its versatility. The door frame is the most obvious item around the house to use but you can also do this stretch on the side of a gym machine, using a TRX or some kind of resistance band, or even a lamppost if you're training outside.

This stretch can feel very similar to the Hanging exercises (page 102) because you have something at the front to grip on to, which creates a really nice sensation of lengthening throughout the body.

HOW TO DO IT...

Start facing a door frame (or the item you are using) and grab the frame at about shoulder height with your left arm, keeping the arm completely straight. There are numerous ways and angles to do this, so feel free to copy the image I have demonstrated but, like the last stretch, the exact position is not essential. There are a ridiculous number of options. Most important, you want to have the feeling of hanging off the frame / post.

Options are as follows:
Both legs straight / one leg straight, one leg bent
Walk the body around to the left / right
Push the hips back / left / right
Take arm higher / lower

Try all of the above angles and see what stretches come up for you. It's a really powerful stretch to get into all kinds of new angles for the sides, back and shoulders, as well as strengthening the arms.

There will definitely be some strength, grip and mobility elements to as essentially you are hanging with one arm, so take your time to build this one up. Relax the head when in the stretch so your left bicep is by your ear and repeat on the opposite side for your chosen time.

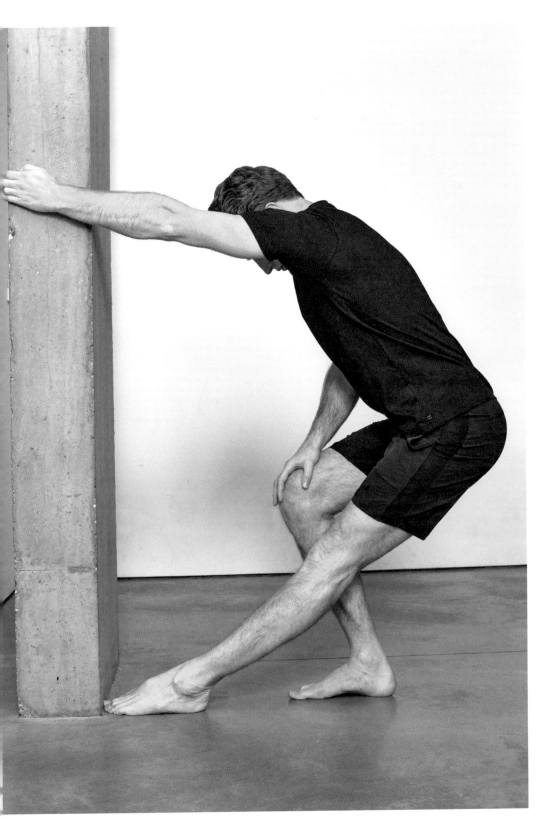

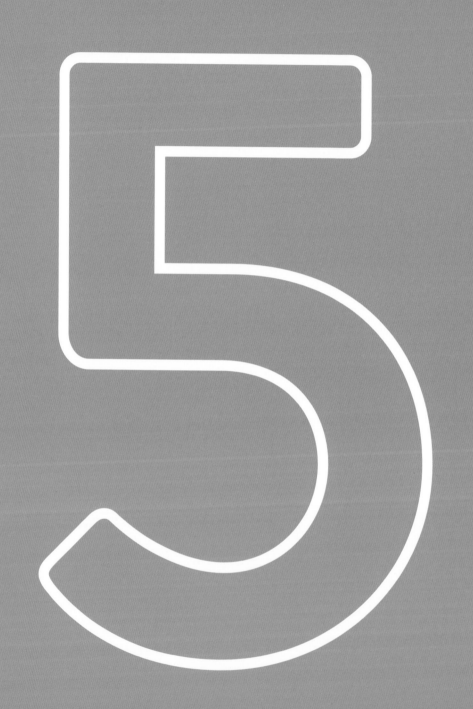

SHOULDERS

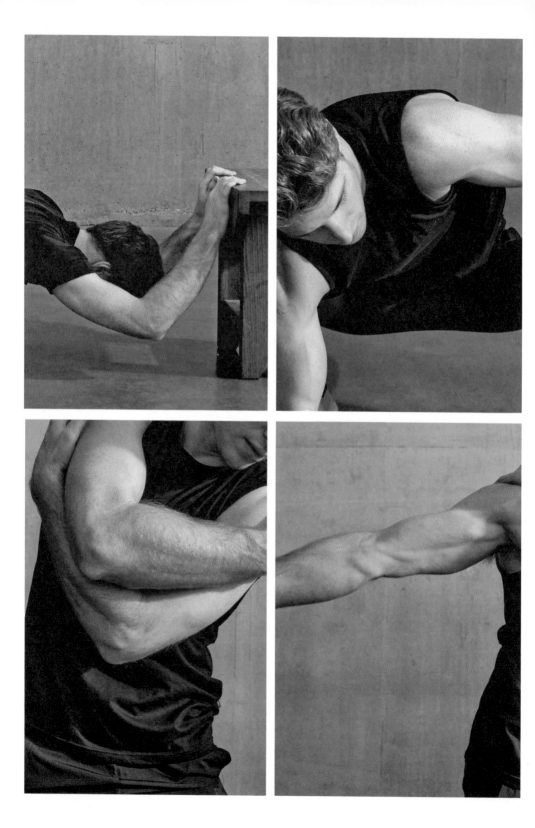

SHOULDERS

Our shoulders often get the most blame for so-called 'bad posture'. Slouchy shoulders are caused by lots of activity in the front of the body – think typing on phones, laptops and computers, coupled with lots of exercises like push-ups, planks and arm strengthening exercises. This is a recipe for pretty tight and immobile shoulders.

Not to worry, the fix is pretty simple – get the shoulders to open in opposing directions; behind the back and over the head. Getting movement back in these two directions will help your shoulders regain a full range of motion.

My shoulder flexibility used to be really bad and the specific strength exercises I performed did not help. I was into bodybuilding and my objective was purely based on aesthetics. I didn't care about the long-term health of my body. All I wanted was to have bigger muscles, especially biceps, triceps, lats and pectorals and I didn't for one second consider the effect this type of training would have on my long-term mobility and range of motion.

Stand up, stand tall, clasp your hands behind your back, straighten your arms and lift them as high as your shoulders.

Only joking! Perhaps even getting your arms straight behind your back with your arms clasped is a hard task here. Now try the opposite: Stand up, stand tall, clasp your hands together in front of your body, straighten your arms above your head and pull the arms back behind your ears as far as you can, sliding your biceps alongside and past your ears. Did your rib cage open? If it did, I want you now to close the rib cage fully and squeeze the buttocks.

If, when making the above adjustments (closing the rib cage and squeezing the butt muscles), you felt the arms come forward, the second and third exercise in this chapter will help you to unlock overhead shoulder flexibility and mobility.

SHOULDERS 1: REVERSE SHOULDER STRETCH

This stretch is a really great shoulder opener and one to do no matter what level of flexibility you are at. It's just an 'instant stretch'. When you do it, I recommend having your hands facing outwards as this will help to stop the elbows from falling out to the sides. If you find the elbows keep falling out to the sides, you can chuck a loop band or a yoga belt around your elbows at first to hold them together at shoulder width.

HOW TO DO IT...

Start sitting on the ground with your knees bent and your feet flat on the floor. If you are using a belt or band, put it around your elbows to stop them falling out to the sides.

Place your hands on the floor behind you, shoulder-width apart, hands facing outwards, and spread your fingers. What you want here is for your elbows to stack above your hands and, at the same time, to get your body as far forwards as you can. You will find, as you take the body forward, the elbows will follow – so, there are two movements going on.

You will need to push your elbows backwards at the same time as taking your body forwards. When doing this, you should feel a stretch in the shoulders, usually the front, and perhaps the back. When in the stretch, you can move left or right with the elbows in order to feel where it is tight and to get deeper into those places. You are working to sit as far forwards as possible, but at the same time always keeping your elbows above the hands.

Quick Tip: Having both your elbows touching a wall behind you can be really helpful. It can help you check that you are even on both sides and is also a good way to keep the elbows in position as you work the body forwards.

Another Quick Tip: Opening the chest in this stretch will help to flatten the back and can be another way to increase and intensify the stretch.

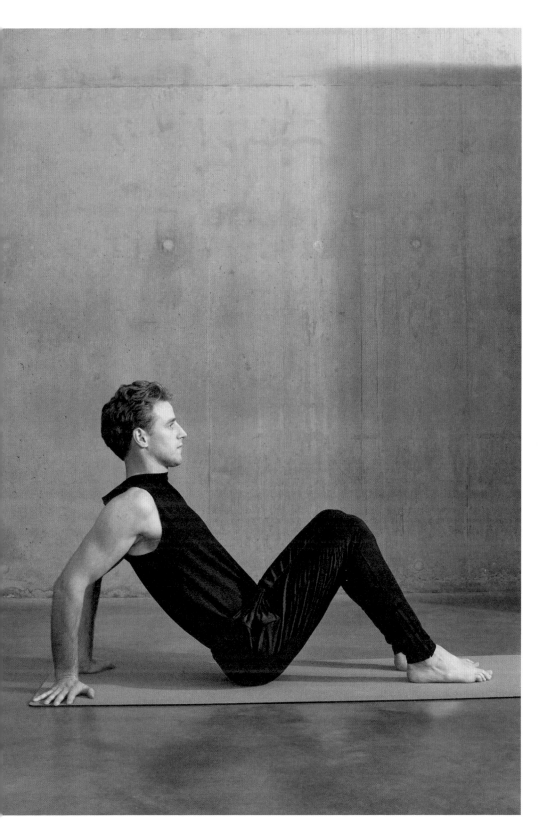

SHOULDERS 2: TABLE HANG

If you don't have a place to hang from at home, don't worry, we have you covered with this hanging variation of a shoulder stretch. Here, I'm using a wooden stall but at home I've used kitchen sides, radiators (please be careful), benches, beds, sofas and tables of all heights. The purpose is the same no matter the object you choose – to lower your armpits towards the ground creating stretches in multiple areas including the lats, triceps, chest, back and shoulders, using your bodyweight as resistance.

The hanging element allows you to relax, or at least to try to relax and I also recommend using a belt or band if you feel your elbows are falling out to the sides. We want to keep the elbows in but without using too much force to pull them in. If we do that, it's going to be difficult to relax.

HOW TO DO IT...

Start kneeling on the ground in front of the object that you are going to be hanging off of, such as a sofa or a small table. Next, grip onto the edge of the surface with your hands around shoulder-width apart. It's a good idea to experiment with the distance here. See where the stretch comes up for you.

Next, relax the armpits down towards the floor – not the head or the chest but the armpits.

Try to think about pushing the elbows forwards and pushing the pelvis backwards at the same time to elongate the body. The result of these two motions will be your armpits lowering towards the ground.

To increase the stretch, take your knees further away from the surface and repeat the above steps. If you find the elbows are falling out the side, use a band or belt to hold them closer in.

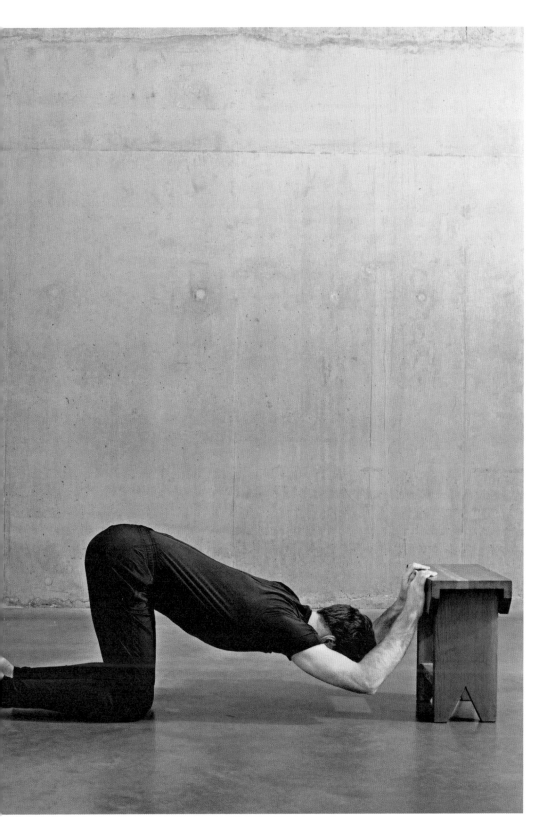

SHOULDERS 3: HANGING (UNDERARM HANG)

We have got to talk about hanging – there is no way I could write a book on essential stretches and not include it. One of the ways I've regained my shoulder health and flexibility is through regular hanging.

When we come across bars in gyms, the first thing that springs to mind is pull-ups or some kind of strength move. What I'm really talking about here is our ability to dead hang. This means using the force of gravity to elongate your body. When you first try this, there is going to be an element of strength involved, particularly as you grip with the hands and arms, but do remember that taking your feet off the floor is not essential.

Now, before you say 'I don't have anywhere to hang from', I just want to let you know that I understand. I am also giving an alternative to hanging (page 92 and page 100) but I have experienced such wonderful benefits from it that it would be a sin for me not to give you the option.

HOW TO DO IT...

Hang on a bar with your feet on the floor and completely relax your shoulders. When you relax your shoulders it should feel almost as if you are pushing the bar up – the distance between your head and the bar will increase as you relax your body down. It's important here that you are hanging and not pulling; this is a relaxing action.

Yes, you will feel some strength element in this stretch but you really want to use the hang to lengthen the body. You will strengthen your grip, your arms and shoulders but you are using the resistance of the body to stretch.

Once you are comfortable hanging for 60 seconds with your feet on the ground, you can work towards doing this exercise with your feet lifted, and then finally in a reverse grip position. This will force your shoulders to rotate externally outwards and introduce more of a stretch in the right direction.

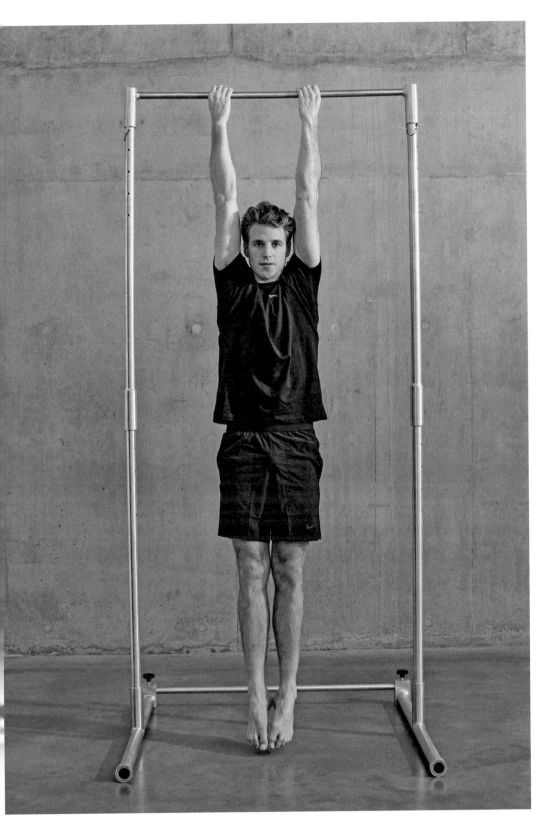

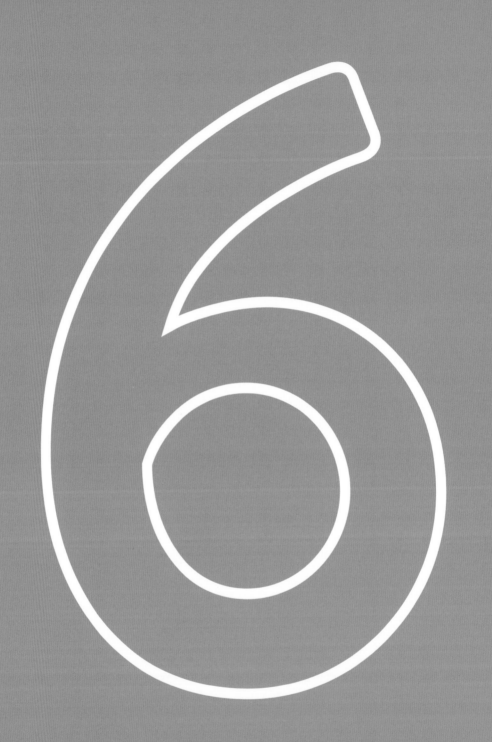

HIPS

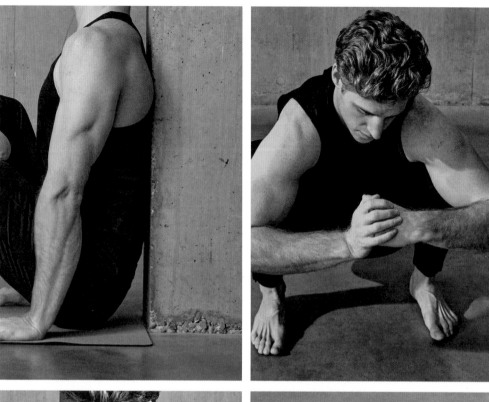

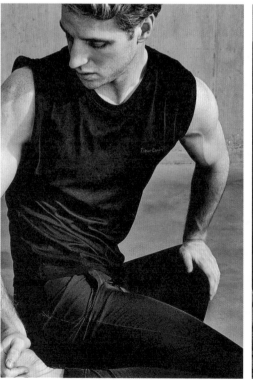

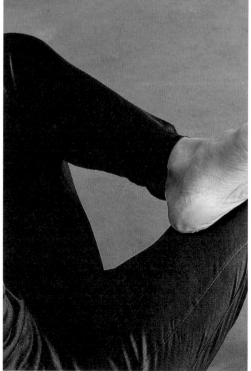

HIPS

The health of our hips defines our ability to function well as we age. Tightness in our hips can affect everyday tasks, including walking or even picking objects up from the ground. Restrictions in the hips inhibit us from performing essential movements. If we don't have full access to our hips then we start to recruit other areas of the body, causing excess strain on our lower back and the knees. These areas are not designed to do the complex movements that the hips are. If we don't keep the hips moving as they should, they become restricted and tight.

Our sedentary lifestyle is the main reason for tightness and a limited range of movement in this part of the body. The second major cause is recreational sports, such as repetitive running and cycling or performing any sport which doesn't include keeping the joints fully mobile or, at the very least, keeping us equally mobile.

Tight hips can wreak havoc on your knees, resulting in shooting pain, lower back pain and parts of the body not functioning as they should. Tightness in the hips also tilts the pelvis out of its natural position, putting unnecessary pressure on the spine.

By following the essential hip movements in this book we will be unlocking tight hips and problem areas, thereby allowing us to sit comfortably on the floor, relax in a squat position, pick things up from the ground safely and get up from the floor without using our hands. All essential movements that we need as we progress through life. This is a slow but rewarding journey that reopens the hips to new levels of movement.

HIPS 1: LAZY WALL STRETCH

This stretch is a genius way to open up the hips with minimal effort. Using the wall makes it very easy to support the body and there are two simple ways to make this stretch easier and more challenging. I recommend doing this on a mat or a grippy surface as there is a tendency to slide away from the wall when in the stretch.

HOW TO DO IT...

Start sitting in your most slouched position (don't worry, we are going to correct this) with your back leaning against a wall and your legs out straight in front of you. Next, bend your right knee so the sole of your right foot is on the floor – you want the sole of the foot to be in contact with the floor at all times as you will use this as leverage. Next, pick up your left foot and place it on your right thigh. For more stretch, place the foot on the thigh, for less lay the ankle on the thigh.

This is your base position. The two adjustments to create more stretch are as follows:

A. Bring the sole of the right foot closer.
B. Sit up taller on the wall.

For maximum stretch over time, work towards getting your lower back closer to the wall. As you progress, focus on lifting the chest up to advance the stretch.

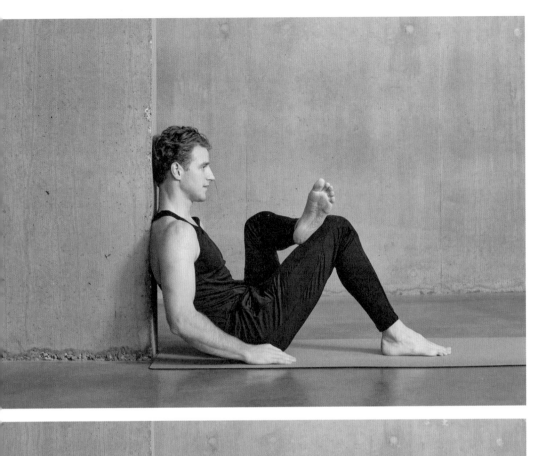

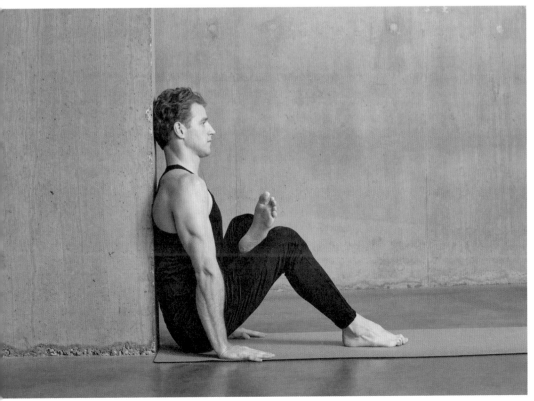

HIP OPENING 2: SINGLE-LEG FROG

If you have previously met Frog (one of the key stretches in *The Flexible Body*), then you should definitely meet its older sibling, Single Leg Frog. There are a couple of key differences to the original Frog and the key one is that you can be much more upright in the position, thereby putting the stretch right where we need to feel it; in the groin.

In this variation you will also benefit from other stretches that may come up, such as all the muscles in the back of the straight leg, especially as we are pushing the sole of the foot against the wall. Because we are upright in the position it's also likely you'll get some stretches in the front of the body; for example, the hip flexor and quad. So, a potential of five different stretches in this movement alone.

HOW TO DO IT...

To begin, kneel on the floor next to a wall. Extend your right leg out until your right foot is flat against the wall, toes pointing up. Grab yourself a block or something soft to put under the knee and also possibly the heel. The last thing you want in this stretch is a knee jamming into the floor.

Once comfortable, and really the key is comfort here, wiggle your knee out as wide as is doable while still remaining upright, as in the image. At this point, you could also hold onto something in front of you, like a chair or a couple of blocks, and build up to placing your hands on the hips. Whichever option you choose, push the hips forward so you feel the buttocks engage. This way the weight will be straight down for maximal stretch.

Your heel and your knee should be in a line.

The foot position of the bent leg can be toes tucked or on your ankle. Again, to avoid any discomfort, you might want to add a mat here.

Stay in the stretch for the given time and change sides once completed. As you progress, the distance between the knee and the opposite heel will increase.

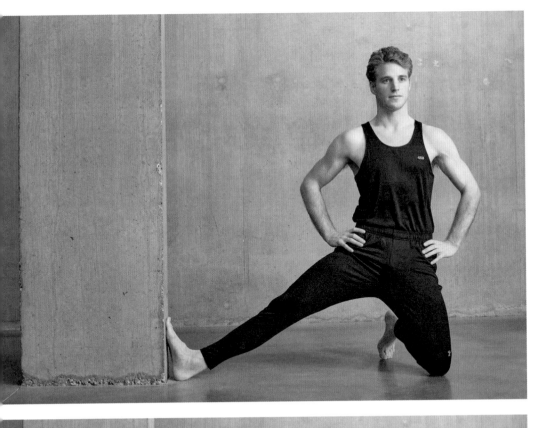

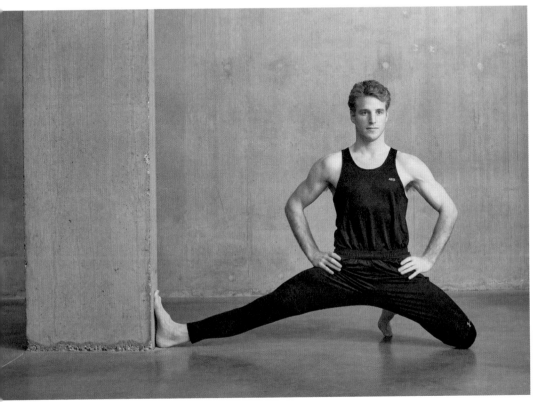

HIP OPENING 3: ELEVATED PIGEON

Elevated Pigeon is one of my favourite stretches as it really allows you to relax in the position whilst, at the same time, creating a really strong stretch. You're unlikely to come across this in a yoga class as these tend not to have benches or somewhere to elevate your leg, but it's very easy to implement at home or at the gym.

In this image I'm using a solid wooden stall with my knee on a concrete surface. This is purely for aesthetics and to make the image look as clear as possible. I recommend you use a softer surface. At home, I use a sofa or a low table with a soft yoga block on top and I always pad up the knee.

As the heights that you might have access to are so varied, the concept of what we are trying to achieve is the most important. Essentially, the higher the surface I use, the more challenging the exercise becomes and the stronger the stretch is going to be.

HOW TO DO IT...

Get into the position you see in the picture as best as you can. Now I'm going to talk through the common issues that might come up. Your raised knee might not lie flat... No problem. Chuck a couple of yoga blocks underneath it – over time it will come lower. Your shin on your back leg might rotate inwards. If it does, it means the hip is rotating out to one side. To combat this, squeeze the buttock of your back leg. By doing this, you'll help to keep the hips square and may also get a bit of a quad / hip flexor stretch on the back leg at the same time. Keep the body upright and try to relax into the position for the given time, before changing over to the other side.

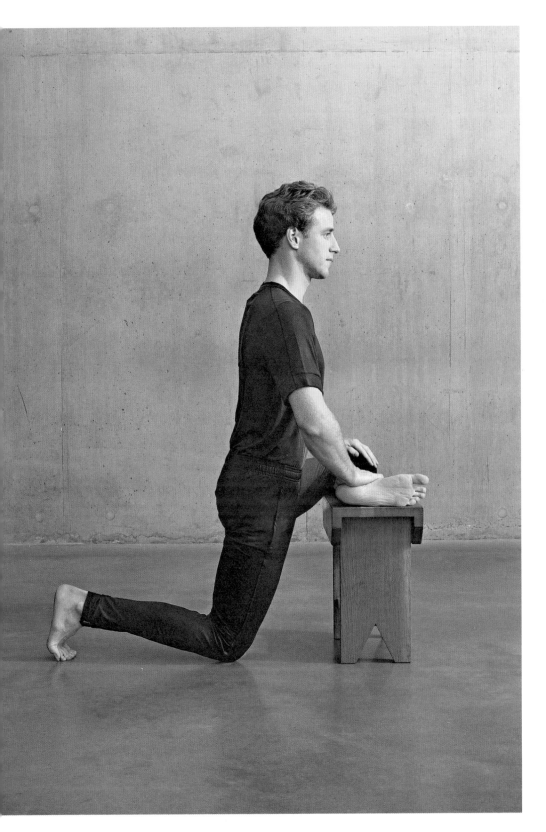

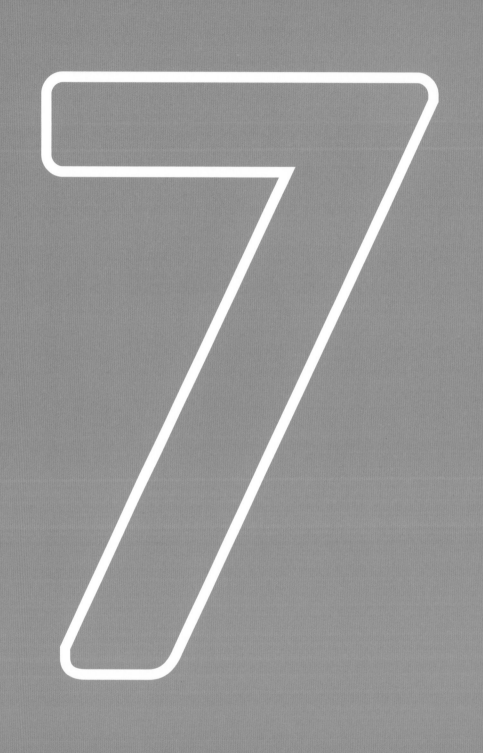

BALANCE

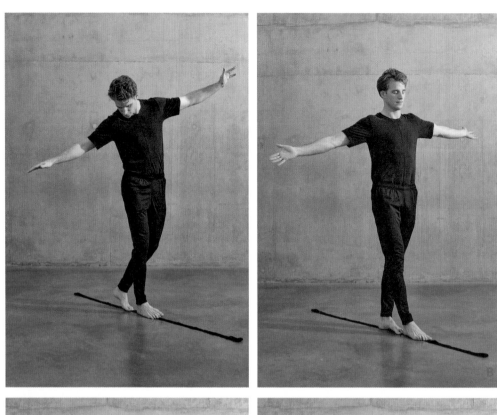

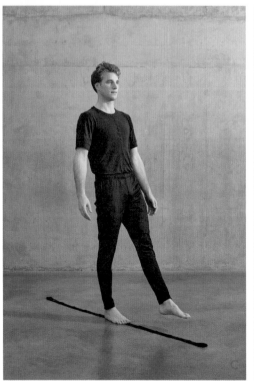
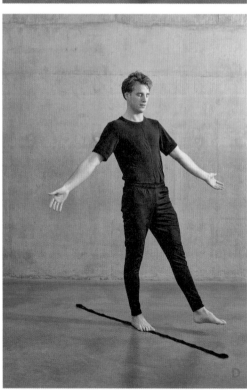

BALANCE

After ticking off the essential movements of the spine, hips and shoulders, the last thing we're going to look at, but certainly not the least important, is balance. Standing on one leg is something we are all capable of doing... until we can't.

Loss of balance is responsible for an incredible number of falls by the elderly each year and the good news is, it's trainable. Balance is essential because, if we can balance, we can walk. Walking is a one-legged exercise; our 10,000 daily steps are all taken on a single leg, albeit for a split second. So practising balancing is like training for walking.

Balance is the lost sense, as Scott McCredie writes in his book *Balance: In Search of the Lost Sense*: 'Losing our sense of balance happens so gradually that you hardly notice it'. Like any form of natural ageing, such as deteriorating vision and hearing, it occurs over many years. However, we have the ability to regain our balance and this can have enormous benefits including, as Scott McCredie writes, 'improved agility, enhanced performance in sports and, for older folks, less chance of falling'.

Having worked with many people aged 65 and over, I've seen first-hand how their balance can improve dramatically by consistently practising and adopting the specific skills in this book. Take my clients, Alexandra and Andreas, for example. They are both 75 years young and they can both now stand on one leg for over a minute. When we started, Alexandra barely managed 10 seconds and used to hold a cane to walk up the stairs. Now, through honing the skill of balance and regular movement, Alexandra just happens to be walking up the stairs unaided. We now use the same cane to stretch her shoulders!

Training balance IS a transferable skill and you'll notice the payoffs in so many other areas – your concentration, your focus and your body's ability to deal with the unexpected. Start slow, know that each time it's working, and repeat! You got this.

BALANCE A: WALK THE LINE

The goal we want to achieve with our balance is to be able to stand on one leg. However, if you are not quite there yet, the key exercise we need to work on is to walk in a straight line. Yes, I'm talking about a sobriety test used for drunk drivers. This tests your balance and coordination, which is exactly what we are doing, except we're also going to mix it up by reversing the process.

This is a practice exercise to get you used to balance before you begin the more challenging exercises. For this, there are two options: walk forwards in a straight line or, for a more advanced variation, walk backwards in a straight line.

For this exercise you will need to have a straight line to follow on the floor. Some good ideas are the edge of a mat, the edge of a rug, the lines of the floorboards if you have wooden floors or placing a piece of tape on the floor. This is something that you're going to be doing every day, so set yourself up with whatever is easy to organize daily.

HOW TO DO IT...

To begin, take your shoes and socks off and place one foot on the line. The whole foot should be pointing forwards and be placed directly over the line. Next, place the other foot directly in front of it and keep going until you have completed your chosen time. For the backwards alternative, do the same thing backwards.

If using a rug, a good idea is to walk around it, placing each step on the edges of the rug.

Note: The steps should be done SLOWLY, and you should be aiming for the least number of steps possible within the time. Really focus on the detail of each step and make sure your feet are facing forward and lift the hands out to the side as much as you need to help you.

BALANCE B: FEET IN FRONT

For the first balance exercise, you are still going to have two feet on the floor, except there is a twist. Not a literal one but you will be attempting this exercise with your eyes closed, so do make sure you are familiar and comfortable with walking in a straight line before moving on to this variation.

Trying any balance exercise with your eyes closed makes it far more challenging. This is because you use your eyes to sense where you are in space. Without this visual help, the body has to respond entirely by feeling the changes in balance rather than being able to see that your balance needs altering to maintain the position. Working on your balance is good for your long-term mobility but, when you practise it with your eyes closed, it also improves your concentration.

HOW TO DO IT...

In the introductory exercise, you were placing one foot in front of the other. For this exercise, you are going to start in the same position, with one foot placed directly in front of the other.

Place one foot in front of the other, get your balance and then slowly close your eyes as you try to stay in the same position. You may feel an instant wobble in one or both of the feet, which may take you by surprise, but build it up over the time. It takes concentration to work on this one.

Your aim is either to complete the exercise for your chosen time with the eyes open or with the eyes closed for a more advanced variation. You want to be able to complete both these exercises for your chosen time before moving on to the One-Legged Stand.

Quick Tip: Leaning forwards onto the front leg, or backwards onto the back leg can really help you find the point of balance. Experiment with both and see what works best for you. You also have the option to put your arms out to the side to assist.

BALANCE C: REGULAR ONE-LEGGED STAND

The second balance exercise is a One-Legged Stand. If at first this feels impossible, you need to spend some more time on your straight-line walking (see page 118). If fear of falling is an issue, have a wall close to you for safety. I always want you to challenge yourself, but I also always want you to feel safe.

Standing on one leg is a great exercise for learning how to put your full bodyweight on one leg, and also encourages focus and concentration. Remember, you want to have balance for life. For some of you, who are perhaps not at an age where you feel it's challenging you, be careful not to rush through this exercise. It's not one to take lightly and to tick off like you've completed it. It needs to be part of your daily training as, if you don't train your balance, before you know it, it will be gone.

HOW TO DO IT...

Start standing tall, feet together, away from any walls (as long as you feel safe). All toes should remain on the ground. Now, as you are going to balance on the right side first, you want to lean the whole body across to the right. If you just keep your right shoulder above your right foot, you will never find the point of balance. However, if you lean to the right then you will start to find the point of balance.

At first, you can use the left foot to help you find that point by pushing your toes into the floor and gently transferring your bodyweight across to the right. Raising the arms out to the side will also help you to find that point of balance.

As you practise this regularly, the goal is to be able to stand on each leg for 1 minute with the standing thigh engaged, the standing butt muscles engaged and your arms resting down by your sides. Engaging the muscles makes sure you are always working to keep the legs and hips strong as opposed to just hinging on the joints. You need your legs to stay strong individually to support you for the rest of your life.

BALANCE D: EYES CLOSED ONE-LEGGED STAND

Have you ever tried balancing on one leg with your eyes closed? Well, if you've mastered the last two exercises, this is what you've arrived at. We have to ask ourselves, what is the purpose of a practice, of training? The purpose is to put us in an extreme position where we are overperforming on the skill we need to master. Let me give you an example:

When you're doing your driving test, the level of perfection and number of points required are far in excess of what it takes to actually be able to drive. It's through regular practice that you become a driver but you first need to take that initial lesson and learn how to overperform under pressure when learning new skills.

Over-prepare your body for what life may bring. We practise balancing with the eyes closed to make sure the body is always overperforming in training for the skills we need in life. This gives us some leeway as we age, some room for error.

The Eyes Closed One-Legged Stand requires mental focus, 100 per cent concentration and lots of practice. It's a skill that we perform at the beginning of every class I teach, whether in person or online.

HOW TO DO IT...

Make sure you are somewhere where you cannot be distracted as you need your full attention for this exercise. First, look down at the foot you are going to balance on. When your eyes are closed you will need to envision that foot in contact with the ground. For example, I've been doing this for so long now that it almost feels as though my eyes are open.

It's a little bit like knowing your room at night when you turn the light off and then suddenly a phone charger has been left on the floor and you stand on it. Ouch, my brain didn't have that in its map.

Once you are fully focused and ready, follow the steps for the Regular One-Legged Stand (page 120) but with the eyes closed. I always suggest you don't squeeze the eyes closed but rather close them softly as though your eyes are open behind the lids. If you've never tried this before it's highly likely you're not going to be able to do it, but over time and with practice you will be able to do it regularly, with the standing thigh and butt engaged and the arms relaxed down by your sides.

Note: In the Closed Eyes One-Legged Balance, your foot will constantly adjust. Don't be disheartened by this. You are doing the exercise correctly. I also suggest setting a timer for your given time beforehand and include an extra 10 seconds for set-up time. Even if you keep coming out of it, keep trying until that timer goes off. Practice makes perfect.

COMMON PROBLEM AREAS

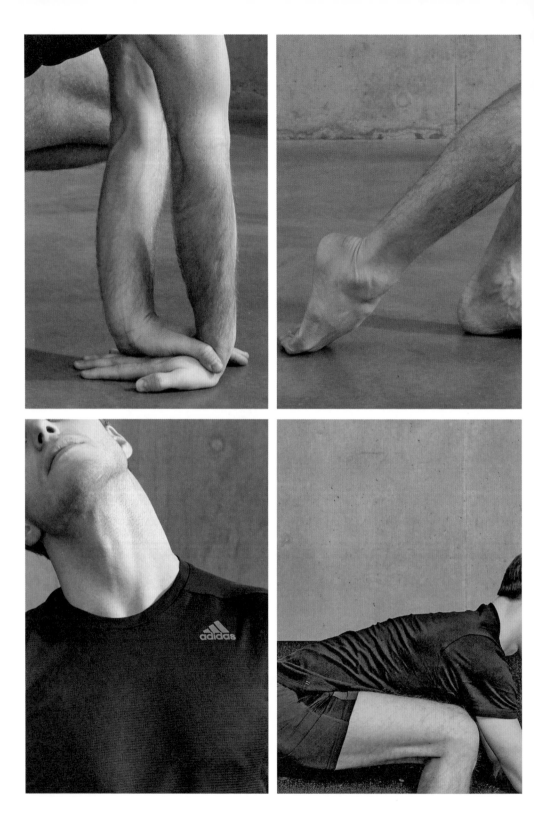

COMMON PROBLEM AREAS

Now we have covered the seven essential stretches it's time to look at some of the most common problem areas. These all concern areas of the body that are bearing the brunt of our tech revolution and so these 15 bonus stretches target specific parts of the body that often get the least amount of attention and frequently present as problem points for many people.

Feet – Our feet tend to spend far too long squeezed into tight, impractical shoes so these foot stretches will reverse the tightness and send a positive chain reaction up through the whole body.

Neck – Often trapped between an inactive upper back and a busy brain, this is our second most vulnerable area of the body when it comes to experiencing pain (after the lower back). The stretches here will lengthen that tight tissue in all directions.

Front of Hips – Hello back pain! Reopening the front of the hips is essential for reversing the long-term effects of repetitive sitting, as well as relieving the extra strain placed on the hips and back.

Shoulder Blades – One of the most ignored areas of the body, but as we get them gliding up, down and around our back, expect a huge relief in neck symptoms, plus the feeling of being lifted upright.

Hands – Most commonly used these days for typing and texting, but evolved for gripping, grasping, pushing, pulling and climbing, it's time to strengthen and lengthen our hands and wrists.

IT Band / Outside of the Leg – Tightness here commonly results in shooting pains down the legs and directly impacts our lower backs. Stretching can only be a good thing.

FEET

Our feet can get tight from shoes, sports and other types of activity. We're so reliant on this essential part of the body and yet we rarely think about stretching it.

A: This stretch is inspired by a yoga exercise called Broken Toe. This single leg variation, which I call the Toe Buster, can be used to discover particularly tight spots. Start in a squat position, stepping your left leg forwards with your knee roughly above your ankle. Make sure to keep your full weight down through your left heel. As you start to lower your right knee towards the floor you should feel a strong stretch through your left toes. I suggest leaning left to right to find the stretch. To make this easier, place a couple of blocks / books underneath your right knee. Over time, and to increase the stretch, take the knee closer to the floor by either lowering it down or reducing the blocks. Repeat on the opposite side.

B: Ever sat in a squat and felt like you're falling backwards? When we opt for chairs instead of our natural sitting position, the squat, the achilles tendon tightens up, so it's important to add these exercises to your routine. Start in a kneeling position and bring your left foot round to the front. Sitting tall, use your hands to push up on your left thigh, bringing your knee over your toes. Swing your back knee to the side, taking it further back as you improve the stretch. You should feel this right in the back of your front foot. Flipping the back foot onto its side will help push the stretch into the right spot. Hold for the given time and switch to the opposite side.

C: This stretch is an advanced version of kneeling on the floor, making sure we work into the front of the ankle. Start in a kneeling position and grab a block or a couple of books, placing them underneath your knees. Keep the torso upright and relax into the stretch making sure the ankles don't collapse out to the sides. If you feel any pain in the knees remove the block.

D: We've already stretched the toes in one direction and now it's time to counter stretch. I recommend doing this stretch on a softer surface like a mat or a carpet. The more weight you put through the leg you're stretching the more you will feel it. Now you're here, start moving the ankles, drawing circles in both directions. Switch legs and repeat on the other side.

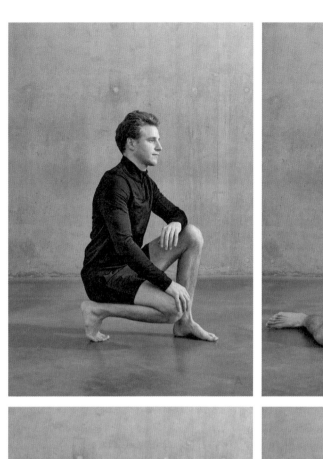

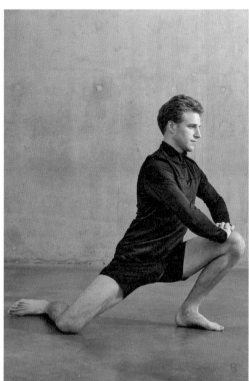

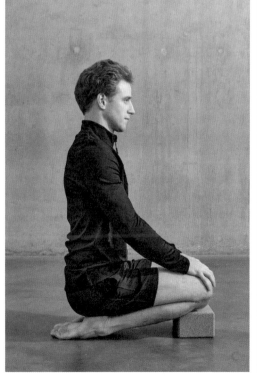

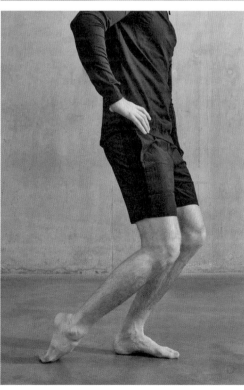

NECK

I've mentioned back and neck pain, so it makes sense to include some specific stretches targeted at the neck, and one that also has an extra shoulder stretch included too. I just want to reiterate that, even though these are neck stretches, it does not mean that they will 'fix' neck pain. Neck, back and other common types of pain are largely referred pain, and it's only by stretching the full body that you will start to see a reduction in pain. Where the pain occurs is not necessarily the specific problem area.

Please go easy with these stretches. As you are taking the hand over the top to lightly pull on the head, be really gentle, and rather guide up and along rather than just yanking your head to the side. Perform them in a position where you can sit up tall, like at your desk or on your sofa.

HOW TO DO IT...
A: Clasp your hands behind your neck and lightly pull your chin to your chest until you feel a light stretch. Try to keep your chest open when doing this and hold for the given time. **Quick Tip:** This stretch can also be done lying on the floor, staring up at the ceiling.

B: Place your right hand on the back of your head. Now turn your chin to face your right armpit. At this point squeeze your left shoulder blade back and down whilst very lightly pulling on the back of the head with your right hand. These two motions will create a neck stretch. Once finished, repeat on the opposite side.

C: Reach your right hand over your head to just above your left ear and slide your left hand across your lower back. Gently pull your right ear to your right shoulder being careful not to yank on the head. At the same time squeeze your left shoulder blade back and down into its socket. Feel free to adjust the height of the chin, in the stretch trying it higher and lower to target different areas. Once finished, repeat on the other side.

D: Lift the chin up in the air whilst simultaneously taking your right ear to the right shoulder, this is similar to stretch three except that, without the hands, you are not limited on the direction you can move in. You might also want to try this with the mouth slightly open when in the stretch. You'll see the effect when you try it. This will help to relieve tension in the jaw. Whilst in the stretch, keep the shoulder blades pulled back and down. Once finished, repeat on the opposite side.

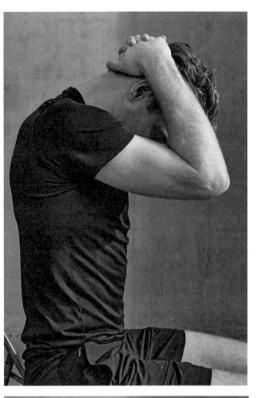
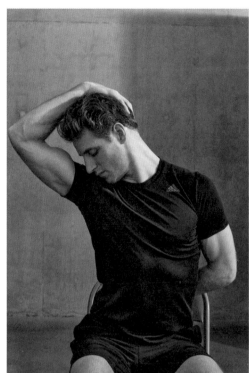
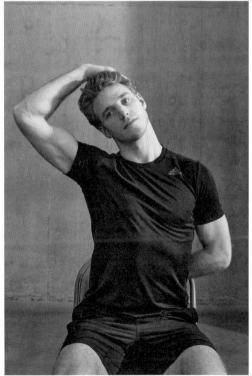
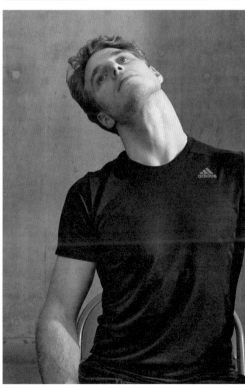

HIP FLEXORS

As sitting has become so prevalent, I wanted to add an extra exercise to target the higher part of the quad / hip flexor area. In fact, a study in 2008, looking at preventing falls in the elderly, showed an improved function in walking, including greater step length, after doing static stretches targeting this particular area of the body. It concluded that stretching exercises targeting the hip flexors were a promising strategy to reduce the risks of falls.

Now, you may or may not be elderly, but the reality is that one day we all hope to be and the likelihood is that, if you're young now, you'll have grown up with massive amounts of sedentary screen-time. Therefore, it's important that you have the tools in place to undo the effects of this.

For this particular exercise, nick-named the Sofa Slider, you need a sofa or a bench – you can see in the pictures that it works really nicely when I'm holding onto the arm of a sofa for support. This helps me to keep my back upright and really open up the front of my hip. Depending on your sofa, you might not have this option; hence we added another.

HOW TO DO IT...
Start on a sofa or bench or a flat surface that is long enough to have your full leg on and high enough so that you can have your right leg hanging over the edge in a lunge position with your right knee roughly above the heel.

When in the stretch, if doing the upright variation (which is the ideal), use your arms to keep the body upright. If you are doing the other, rest your elbows on the surface. In either position, be careful of the right knee (the one in the lunge) drifting out to the outside as this will take the stretch off. Once you have completed your time, repeat on the other side.

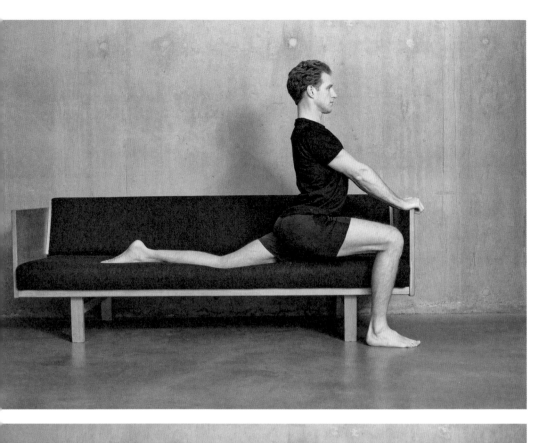

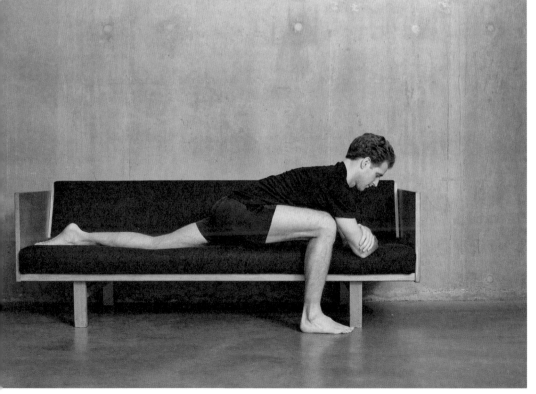

SHOULDER BLADES

I don't think there is any exercise quite like this one and I really believe it's deserving of its place here due to the amount of time we spend on our phones, laptops etc. Being static, no matter the position, makes the tissue around our upper backs very tight. A great way to loosen up this tissue and free your shoulder blades is with Scapular Squeezes. The most effective way to do this is with your hands on the floor or a flat surface so you can use it to push against.

The movement in the exercise is not, I repeat NOT, coming from the arms. In this exercise, your arms do nothing. Well, at least that is the plan. If it's challenging to keep your elbows straight at first, don't worry, this will come and, as you practise it more, you will start to feel the movement really coming through the shoulder blades. The straighter you can keep the arms, the more movement will be coming through the shoulder blades.

HOW TO DO IT...

Start on all fours on the floor with your shoulders directly above your wrists, your hips roughly above your knees and your hands facing outwards. Without leading with the head, aim to keep the arms straight and tap the shoulder blades together. Be careful here not to squeeze the shoulder blades up into the neck but rather aim down towards the middle of your back – so it's together and down. To separate the shoulder blades, first re-straighten the elbows and push tall into the floor. Keep moving slowly through these two positions, working in this order: straighten elbows, squeeze shoulder blades back and down, straighten elbows, push tall. As you progress with this you'll need fewer reminders to keep your elbows straight.

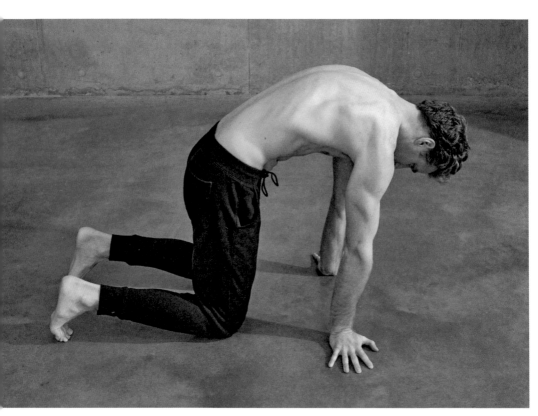

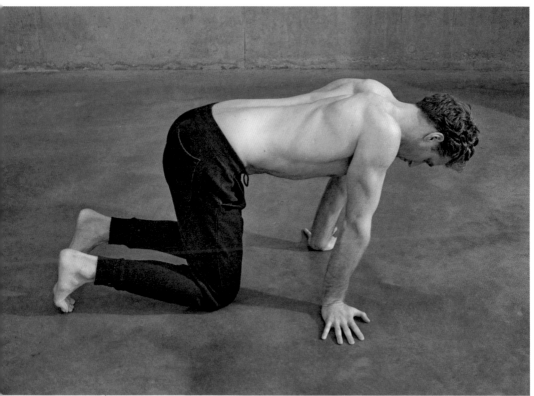

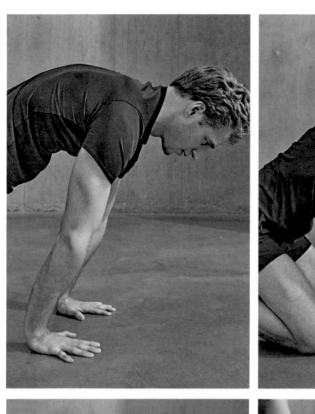
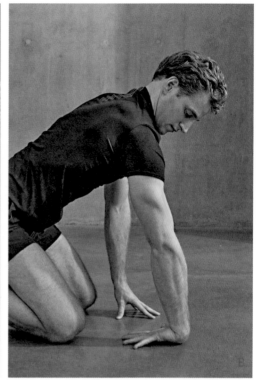
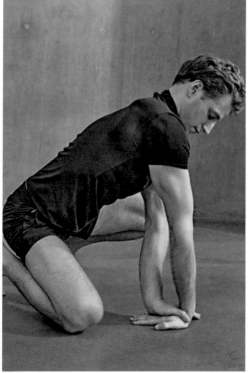
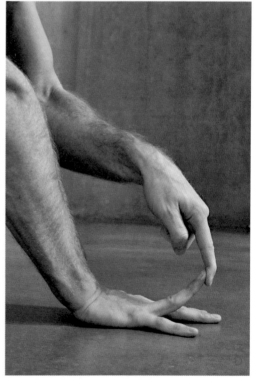

HANDS

With all of these stretches I suggest kneeling on the floor on a comfortable mat or carpeted surface so you are comfortable enough to fully focus on the stretches. You can either hold the stretches or move slowly in them. Back off if you feel any wrist pain. Just pure stretch only.

HOW TO DO IT...

A: Spread your fingers and place both of your hands on the floor around shoulder-width apart with the fingers facing forwards. Press the heel of the hands down into the floor and lean forwards slightly, keeping the elbows straight until you feel a stretch. There are options here to either hold in the position, move backwards and forwards or draw circles in both directions.

B: Turn your right palm upwards with your fingers facing you, then place the back of this hand on the ground, spread your fingers and aim to straighten your arm. I say aim; this may feel a little tight at first. Either work over time towards straightening the arm or, if you can get the elbow straight, your options here are either to hold in the position, move backwards and forwards or draw small wrist circles. Repeat on the opposite side once your time is up.

C: Place your palm on the floor with your fingers facing towards you. Spread your fingers and push the heel of your hand into the ground. Now, slowly rock backwards and forwards with the hips, aiming to get your hips closer to your heels over time. When in the stretch, either hold, rock slowly or draw circles into the ground. As your flexibility improves, take your knees further back and repeat the above steps. Don't forget the other side.

D: Place one of your palms down on the floor with the fingers facing away from you. Now start the clock. Throughout the time, lift up each finger and thumb off the floor in turn whilst keeping the palm of the hand in firm contact with the surface. You can either pull directly upwards or draw small circles. Spend around 10 seconds on each digit as you move through the time and then repeat on the other side.

IT BAND

I promise I'm not posing! You know, I actually came across this stretch
by accident when playing around with a One-Legged Balance exercise
variation. Normally, to stretch this area I like to lie on the floor with a belt
around my foot and use that to manoeuvre stretch into the outside of my
leg but this one is actually pretty simple to get into. It requires minimal
equipment and really hits the spot. I'm also going to talk you through a few
equipment options below that will come in handy as variants for this specific
stretch. In the image, as you can see, I'm using a block. However, you might
want to replace this block with a chair, a sofa, a table, or anything that
brings your torso higher so you're not as deep in the stretch. If you have
more flexibility then of course fingertips on floor, palms on floor, and
then some.

It's quite easy to get this one the wrong way around and I have a habit
of mixing my left and right as I'm teaching this stretch so right now I'm
literally standing up ready to go into this stretch so I can talk you through
it – wish me luck!

HOW TO DO IT...
Ok, firstly stand up with your feet around hip-width apart and your feet
facing forwards. If you're using one, have a block in your hands to the ready.
If you're using an alternative support, place this next to you on your left
hand side.

Next, step your left foot behind you and across to the left. Your left foot is
now behind you, on your right hand side.

Still with me? Ok, good. Now twist your torso to the left so that your hands
are now either on the object you placed there or the block is touching the
floor. Our hands should be on the inside or heading towards the inside of
our right foot.

You can see how easy it is to confuse this one. However, the good thing
is you'll know when you've got it. You'll feel quite a strong stretch on the
outside of your right leg. Take your time with it. As you improve in the
stretch, you'll take your hands lower to the floor or you can just stay on the
surface you are using and bend the elbows to get lower like I am in the image.

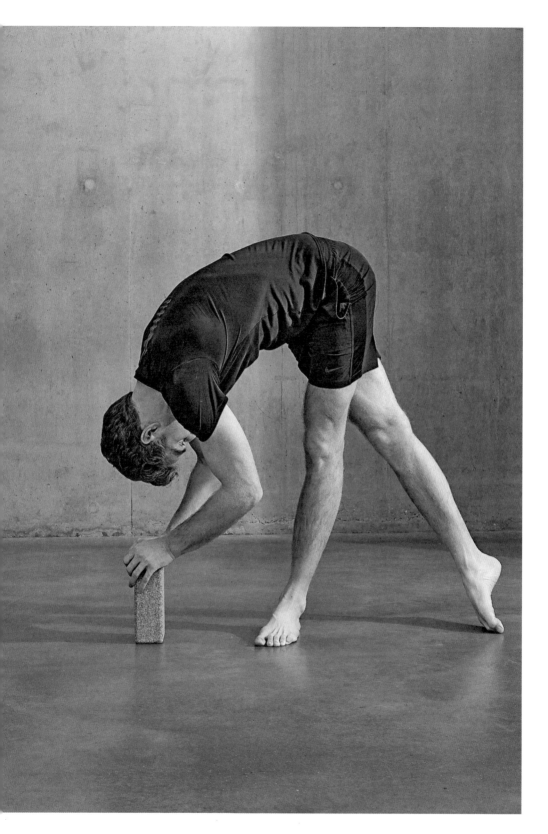

INDEX

RESOURCES

WEBSITES:
www.roger.coach
This is the hub of The Frampton Method. You can find everything here, including our social media pages, latest events, workshops and more.

EQUIPMENT:
So, I mention blocks, books, bands, broomsticks and straps throughout the book. At the time of writing this we've yet to open our Stretch Store. When it is open, you'll find everything you need in this book on my website. Otherwise I recommend typing 'Yoga Block' or 'Yoga Mat' into a search engine and choosing something to suit you.

Alternatively, if you don't want to spend any money, you can of course use a book instead of a block, a couple of towels instead of a mat and a belt instead of a strap.

MY TED TALK 'WHY SITTING DOWN DESTROYS YOU':
https://bit.ly/3jYvFAB
Perhaps you just grabbed this book from the shelf at your local bookstore or came across it online and don't really know much about my backstory or why I'm all about stretching. My TED talk, aptly named 'Why Sitting Down Destroys You', has been viewed, at the time of writing, by over 3 million people. If you'd like to watch the 13-minute talk where I discuss my childhood idol, you can find this on YouTube.

APPS:
I mention the many benefits of hanging throughout the book: the app **Calisthenics Parks** is a great resource for finding local parks and outdoor gyms near you.

BOOKS:
The Flexible Body – Roger Frampton, Pavilion (2018)

ACKNOWLEDGEMENTS

I've never had many close friends in my life but when you have a whole entourage of siblings, each with their unique and powerful personalities, why would you need to?! Love you Mum, Dad, Freddie, Gloria, David, Joel, Jane, Phoebe and Peter. Life would not be the same without you! Love you forever guys!

All my love to my partner Izzy and our little woof woof Alan. It's not easy living with Benjamin Button you know! The older I get, the more sofas, chairs and tables rapidly turn into stretch weapons and movie nights into squat practice.

Huge, huge thanks to my not-just-manager but good friend Francesca Zampi, for working alongside me on the concept for this book and, would you believe it... her fashion photographer husband Jesse John Jenkins for pulling out the stops in a shut-up-shop 2020 London and shooting this book. And, as always, a huge thanks to the team at Pavilion for believing in my message and pushing me to spread my message!

To the two people who have had the biggest impact on my life... Dominic Richards and Brian Rose. If it weren't for you both, I'd never have started this journey to begin with. Thank you, from the bottom of my heart!

And last, but by no means the least, I really want to acknowledge you, the reader, for making the time to read this book and taking a HUGE action step in your life.

I've met many parents who say that there comes a time in your life when things stop being about you, and life becomes about your kids and those you love. Watching people's movement change and the improvement in their bodies, I really get that feeling now. I started off on my journey with all these huge goals of how I'm going to do this with my body and that with my body and it was really all about me. But that true magical feeling comes when we get those little messages from the readers saying how much this book has impacted on their life.

... and that is real gold dust! Thank you.

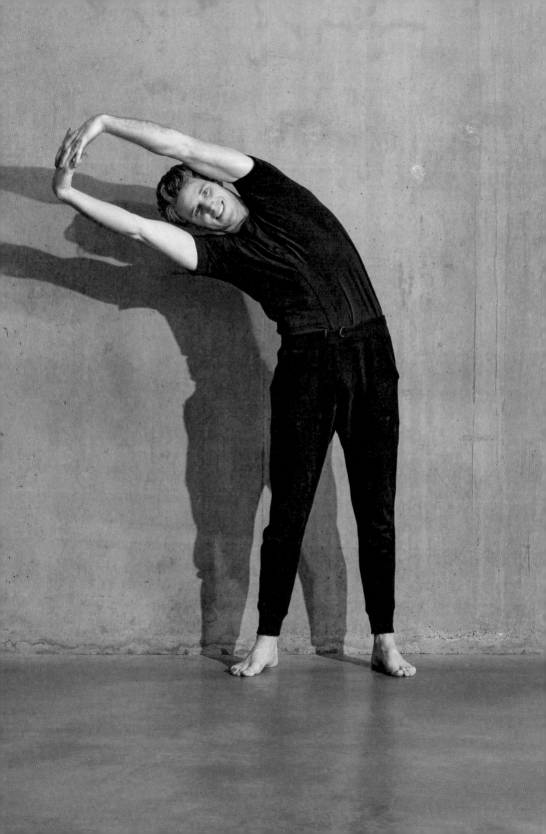

ABOUT ROGER

Roger Frampton is a Movement Coach specializing in functional performance and is the creator of the Frampton Method.

His revolutionary training techniques place emphasis on conscious movement. He combines bodyweight exercises with aspects of gymnastics and yoga to help us better understand the natural functionality of our bodies, with the aim of preventing pain and returning us to the fluid way we moved as children.

Viewed over 3 million times, Roger's TED Talk, 'Why Sitting Down Destroys You', explores his theory that modern sedentary office life has created a myriad of problems for people's strength and flexibility. Furthermore, he believes that the fitness industry and its focus on punishing exercise routines does little to counteract this. His book, *The Flexible Body*, offers mindful movement solutions to do at home and has been an Amazon bestseller several times since it was published in January 2018.

The Frampton Method has been featured in; *The Sunday Times*, *Grazia*, *Esquire*, *Elle*, *Men's Health* and *GQ* and Roger has appeared on *Sky News*, *BBC Business* and *Virgin Radio*.

Prior to qualifying as a professional coach, Roger worked as an international model for over a decade, appearing in ad campaigns for Ralph Lauren, Orlebar Brown and Aquascutum.

First published in the UK in 2021 by
Pavilion
43 Great Ormond Street
London
WC1N 3HZ

ISBN: 9781911663881

A CIP catalogue record for this book is
available from the British Library.

10 9 8 7 6 5 4 3 2 1

Reproduction by Rival Colour Ltd., London
Printed and bound by IMAK Offset, Turkey

www.pavilionbooks.com

Publisher: Helen Lewis
Editor: Cara Armstrong
Copyeditor: Vicky Orchard
Design manager: Laura Russell
Photographer: Jesse John Jenkins
Photographer's assistant: Betty Martin
Illustrations: Bárbara Malagoli
Production controller: Phil Brown